STUTTERING

REMEDIATION OF COMMUNICATION DISORDERS SERIES
Frederick N. Martin, Series Editor

STUTTERING

_____ *Edward G. Conture*

HEARING IMPAIRMENTS IN YOUNG CHILDREN

_____ *Arthur Boothroyd*

HARD OF HEARING CHILDREN IN REGULAR SCHOOLS

Mark Ross with Antonia Maxon
_____ *and Diane Brackett*

HEARING-HANDICAPPED ADULTS

_____ *Thomas G. Giolas*

ACQUIRED NEUROGENIC DISORDERS

_____ *Thomas P. Marquardt*

LANGUAGE DISORDERS IN PRESCHOOL CHILDREN

_____ *Patricia R. Cole*

LANGUAGE DISORDERS IN SCHOOL AGE CHILDREN

_____ *Mary Lovey Wood*

Forthcoming

ARTICULATION DISORDERS

_____ *Ronald K. Sommers*

CEREBRAL PALSY

_____ *James C. Hardy*

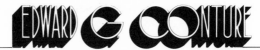

EDWARD G. CONTURE

Syracuse University

STUTTERING

Prentice-Hall, Inc., Englewood Cliffs, New Jersey 07632

Library of Congress Cataloging in Publication Data

Conture, Edward G.
   Stuttering.

   (Remediation of communication disorders)
Bibliography: p.
Includes index.
1. Stuttering. I. Title. II. Series.
RC424.C575   616.85'54   81-7387
ISBN 0-13-858977-1   AACR2

© 1982 by Prentice-Hall, Inc., Englewood Cliffs, N.J. 07632

616.8554
C756s

Printed in the United States of America

10 9 8 7 6 5 4 3 2 1

Editorial production/supervision by Virginia Cavanagh Neri
Interior design by Maureen Olsen
Cover design by Maureen Olsen
Manufacturing buyer: Edmund W. Leone

Prentice-Hall International, Inc., *London*
Prentice-Hall of Australia Pty. Limited, *Sydney*
Prentice-Hall of Canada, Ltd., *Toronto*
Prentice-Hall of India Private Limited, *New Delhi*
Prentice-Hall of Japan, Inc., *Tokyo*
Prentice-Hall of Southeast Asia Pte. Ltd., *Singapore*
Whitehall Books Limited, *Wellington, New Zealand*

TO ED AND HELEN

#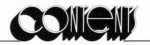

Foreword xi

Preface xiii

Introduction 1

AN ORIENTATION 2
objective, behavioral descriptions 3   psychosocial as
well as physiological aspects 3   stutterers as people
and as individuals 4   rationales versus recipes 5
problem solving versus the program 6

WHAT IS STUTTERING?: PERCEPTUAL
CONSIDERATIONS 7

WHAT IS STUTTERING?: PHYSIOLOGICAL
CONSIDERATIONS 11

WHO IS A STUTTERER? 15

SOME PARTING THOUGHTS 17

SUMMARY 18

Evaluation 19

A FEW WORDS REGARDING THE EQUIPMENT USED IN
EVALUATING STUTTERING 21

COMPONENTS OF THE STUTTERING EVALUATION 22
the intake form 22   the interview procedure 23

ASSESSING COMMUNICATIVE AND RELATED BEHAVIOR
DURING THE STUTTERING EVALUATION 28
fluency 28   hearing 30   voice 30   articulation 32
language 33   reading 33   intelligence 33
neuromuscular 35   psychological 35

WHO IS AND WHO IS NOT REFERRED FOR THERAPY 37

SUMMARY 39

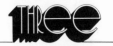

Remediation: young children who stutter 40

YOUNG CHILDREN WITH NO COMMUNICATIVE
CONCERNS, WHOSE PARENTS ARE CONCERNED 44

CHILDREN WITH SOME STUTTERING AND
(UN)CONCERNED PARENTS 47

CHILDREN WHO CLEARLY STUTTER AND PARENTS WHO
ARE (UN)CONCERNED 55

REFERRALS TO OTHER PROFESSIONALS 64

GENERAL SUGGESTIONS REGARDING PARENT
COUNSELLING 65

SUMMARY 67

Remediation: older children and teenagers who stutter 69

INTRODUCTION 70

OLDER CHILDREN WITH MINIMAL OR LITTLE AWARENESS
OF STUTTERING 72
  desensitization 74   ignoring the child: a potent but
  difficult to discern fluency disruptor 76

THE OLDER CHILD DIFFERS FROM THE YOUNGER
CHILD 77
  encouraging the child to (non)verbally interact with
  peers 78   the gradual process of learning or
  learning about learning 79

OLDER CHILDREN WITH DEFINITE AWARENESS OF
STUTTERING 79
  motivation 80   identification 81   modification 82
  parent's role in remediation 85   (dis)continuing
  therapy 86   making changes in speech 87
  encouraging the child to talk 89   practice 89

TWELVE- TO FOURTEEN-YEAR-OLD STUTTERERS:
TURNING THE CORNER INTO ADOLESCENCE 90
  description 90   factors to consider 93   when to
  begin and when not to begin therapy 96   objectively
  changing speech behavior 96   motivating client to
  make speech changes 98   practice and/or
  carryover of change 99   difficulties gauging changes
  in speech 101   related concerns: academics, social
  life, and employment 101

SOME PARTING THOUGHTS 105

SUMMARY 106

Remediation: adults who stutter 107

INTRODUCTION 108

PROBLEM DICTATES PROCEDURE 109

GROUP AND/OR INDIVIDUAL THERAPY 110

INDIVIDUAL THERAPY WITH ADULTS WHO STUTTER:
FIRST IMPRESSIONS 113
  after first impressions 113   identification 114   I'm
  beginning to stutter more 120   the bridge between
  identification and modification 121   if identification
  fails to develop 122   modification: beginning
  considerations 122   modification: where and what to
  begin changing 123   modification: after then during
  the instance of stuttering 125   modification: when
  the client fails to change 126   modification: when
  the client produces real change 127

WITHIN-THERAPY CARRYOVER 128

CHANGING SPEECH IN CONVERSATION 130

HOMEWORK WITH ADULTS WHO STUTTER 131

SPEECH SHOULD BE AUTOMATIC OR WHY DO I HAVE TO
THINK ABOUT IT ALL THE TIME? 131

WHEN TO DISMISS 133

FOLLOW-UP THERAPY SESSIONS 134

SOME PARTING THOUGHTS 135

SUMMARY 136

Conclusions 138

ORIENTATION 139

EVALUATION PRECEDES REMEDIATION 139

IDENTIFICATION 141

MODIFICATION 142

THE COMMON DENOMINATORS OF STUTTERERS'
THERAPEUTICALLY INDUCED FLUENCY 145

THE CLINICIAN 148

FUTURE DIRECTIONS 150

SUMMARY 152

Appendix 153

A QUESTIONS TO BE ASKED DURING INTERVIEW OF
   THE PARENT(S) OF A DISFLUENT CHILD 154

B THE ONSET OF STUTTERING: A CASE STUDY 158
   introduction 158   procedure 159   the interview 159
   discussion 161

C NOTE TO A BEGINNING SPEECH-LANGUAGE
   PATHOLOGIST 164
   clinicians as people 164   a clinician's need to be
   self-analytical 164   a personality "suitable" for
   becoming a clinician 165   the development of a
   clinician: from classroom to clinic 167   how much
   training you have had 169   "my child's been with
   you for three months and I don't see any change" 170

References 171

Index 180

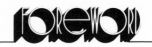

With the information explosion of recent years there has been a proliferation of knowledge in the areas of scientific and social inquiry. The speciality of communicative disorders has been no exception. While two decades ago a single textbook or "handbook" might have sufficed to provide the aspiring or practicing clinician with enlightenment on an array of communication handicaps, this is no longer possible—hence the decision to prepare a series of single-author texts.

As the title implies, the emphasis of this series, *Remediation of Communication Disorders,* is on therapy and treatment. The authors of each book were asked to provide information relative to anatomical and physiological aspects of each disorder, as well as pathology, etiology and diagnosis to the extent that an understanding of these factors bears on management procedures. In such relatively short books this was quite a challenge: to offer guidance without writing a "cookbook;" to be selective without being parochial; to offer theory without losing sight of practice. To this challenge the series' authors have risen magnificently.

Dr. Edward G. Conture comes to the area of stuttering with much first-hand knowledge of what it is like to be the recipient of speech remediation, since both he and his son were born with bilateral clefts of the lip and hard and soft palates. In addition to surgery, both underwent extensive and intensive speech therapy. Dr. Conture, therefore, has a deep, personal appreciation for patients and parents of patients with communicative and related disabilities. His expertise in stuttering has been expanded through his considerable research in this area, much of which has been funded through university, foundation, and federal grants. For more than a decade his active and routine involvement with hundreds of stutterers and their families, along with his knack for cogent and understandable writing, make Dr. Conture an ideal person to write a book on remediation of this most perplexing and misunderstood disorder.

FREDERICK N. MARTIN
Series Editor

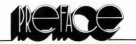

Writing a book on as complex a problem as stuttering, a problem that has resisted solution from some of the best minds in the field of communicative disorders, is indeed a humbling experience. All too quickly, this writer became aware of areas he thought he or least some one else understood only to find out that no one really does! Nevertheless, the many years of speech-language pathologists' research and clinical experience with stuttering have uncovered and established much that is substantial with regard to the remediation of stuttering. Presenting such substantive issues is not always easy, particularly in a text with an applied, clinical orientation, but the author has tried to touch on many such issues. Most of all he has tried not to give this book the appearance of a simplistic solution to a complex problem.

This book is intended for graduate-level student clinicians as well as beginning clinicians in speech-language pathology who are evaluating and remediating stuttering. In these pages the author has tried to strike a balance between formal, scholarly documentation, and less formal clinical experiences, as a basis for discussing the remediation of stuttering. He has also tried to balance a presentation between the stutterer as a stutterer and the stutterer as a human being; that is, he has attempted to balance our orientation between viewing a child, teenager, or adult as a human first and as a stutterer second. Hopefully, he has been relatively successful in striking such balances.

○ ACKNOWLEDGMENTS

The writer of this book owes much to past teachers, colleagues, and family; however, the writer accepts full responsibility for the text and attributes whatever mistakes it may contain totally to himself. Mention of specific past professors will surely result in the exclusion of some, but it is clear to the writer that his education experiences at Emerson College, Northwestern University, and the University of Iowa provided the platform upon which he has been able to construct his professional career. Noteworthy among the writer's many helpful professors were G. Canter, A. Compton, J. Curtis, I. Gormeazano, H. Gregory, J. Hardy, A. Harris, J. Peckham, E. Ward, H. Westlake, and last, but clearly far from least, his mentor, Dean E. Williams. He also thanks past and present Syracuse University colleagues who listened to his ideas, seemingly understood why he would say in effect "I vant to be alone" to write this book, and who have made useful suggestions along the way. Of particular note among these colleagues are B. Blatt, K. Butler, E. Cudahy, S. James, J. McNutt, J. Mills, and J. Saxman. Likewise, the many secretaries who have typed this and earlier drafts have been most helpful. The author extends his appreciation to the many Syracuse University students he has taught and, in turn, learned from. Clearly, these students' questioning of the writer's own understanding of stuttering has induced him to elaborate upon and refine such understanding.

To the writer's parents, Edward and Helen Conture, whose early guidance, love, and strength made everything possible, these notes are of small recompense, but he hopes that they can be taken as some small token of appreciation and love. My wife Shelley, son Brendan, and daughter Tara have been there when it counted, shared the agony as well as the ecstasy, and by asking for little in return have made the author realize he could ask for little more. Finally, he wants to acknowledge the stutterers, their families, and friends, whom he has evaluated and remediated over the years and from whom he has gained so many insights into the problem of stuttering, the world around him, and, most certainly, ourself. Preparation of this manuscript was supported in part by a NINCDS grant (NS 14351) and NINCDS contract (NO1-NS-O-2331) to Syracuse University.

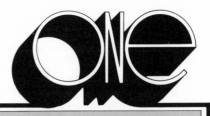

○ AN ORIENTATION

  objective, behavioral descriptions

  psychosocial as well as physiological
  aspects

  stutterers as people and as individuals

  rationales versus recipes

  problem solving versus *the program*

○ WHAT IS STUTTERING?: PERCEPTUAL
  CONSIDERATIONS

○ WHAT IS STUTTERING?: PHYSIOLOGI-
  CAL CONSIDERATIONS

○ WHO IS A STUTTERER?

○ SOME PARTING THOUGHTS

○ SUMMARY

Introduction

○ AN ORIENTATION

Discussing the remediation of stuttering is a bit like discussing the remediation of the common cold. Many "remedies" exist for both stuttering and the common cold, with each remedy being backed by various forms of evidence. Some professionals advocate one form of remediation while others support different forms with equal enthusiasm. To some, the terms *common cold* and *stuttering* represent catchalls for a number of related but different problems with differing causes. Others support the notion that common colds or stuttering have unitary symptoms and causes. Just as folk wisdom suggests that chicken soup helps people with colds, similar wisdom suggests that stutterers may be helped by instructing them to "slow down, take a deep breath, and think about what you're saying." Wherever the truth lies, considered opinion suggests that we are not yet at the point where we can meaningfully discuss curing most peoples' common cold or stutterers' stuttering. Cures, outside those applied to hams and other edibles, suggest total and complete recovery—something a bit short of a miracle, but nevertheless a remarkable event. While we cannot categorically deny the present existence of a cure for stuttering, it seems far more appropriate at this point in time to discuss our abilities, as speech pathologists, to facilitate positive change in the speech and related aspects of individuals who stutter. My purpose in writing this book is not to discuss a cure for stuttering.

My purpose in writing this book is to share approaches to the remediation of stuttering that have been found useful, the rationale and/or reason for their usefulness, and the relative success and failure of these approaches. This should not be considered a "how-to" book; rather, it might more appropriately be called a "this is what needs to be considered" book. We present concepts, ideas, notions, procedures, and strategies that we believe pertinent to consider in the remediation of stuttering. We make no claim that readers of these pages will develop instant expertise or success in the remediation of stuttering. We think, however, that this book provides both the student-clinician and the practicing speech-language pathologist with meaningful insights into some of the more important aspects to consider in the remediation of stuttering. With these thoughts in mind, let me present my general orientation to the clinical management of stuttering.

objective, behavioral descriptions

To begin, we are oriented to consider the problem of stuttering in behavioral terms. We are not referring here to behavioral approaches restricted to this or that school of learning psychology (see Reynolds 1968; Lefrancois 1972; Hill 1977, for overviews of learning psychology). Instead, we are using *behavioral* in the sense of being observable, clearly describable, measurable, and subject to empirical testing within the clinic or experimental setting. We are interested in describing, both for our client and ourself, the client's stuttering problem (both its speech and nonspeech aspects) in as descriptive, objective, and behavioral terms as possible. We consider the client's psychosocial concerns, emotions, and feelings as part of the descriptive territory. Our ability to clearly describe stuttering has a profound influence on our ability to remediate it (Johnson 1946; Williams 1957).

We should strive to describe our client's speech as well as related behavior, for example, expressive language usage, in a fashion that indicates to both ourselves and those we talk to that we know what we are talking about. We are in some state of clinical confusion when we tell our client, "You stutter because you're nervous," or "You are nervous because you stutter." What do we mean by nervous? How do we know that *nerves*, whatever we mean by this term, causes stuttering? For that matter, what do we mean by the word *stuttering*? Obviously, we may push this descriptiveness of language to absurdity by asking, "What do you mean by 'what do you mean'?" Short of such absurdity, we need to realize that our clinical substance (knowledge and activities) is importantly related to our clinical form (language we employ). Johnson (1946) and others have said before that one's language cannot be very clear and of assistance to our clients if our language is not very clear. Our clients will have trouble understanding their stuttering problem (not to mention our therapy) if we state these issues in high levels of verbal confusion.

psychosocial as well as physiological aspects

Also inherent in my orientation to stuttering is a belief in the necessity of understanding the psychosocial as well as the physiological aspects of the problem. It is inappropriate to deal with the disturbed speech physiology associated with stuttering (see Adams 1974; Freeman 1979) without regard for the psychosocial or emotional components of stuttering and vice versa. It is necessary to consider both the psyche (see Sheehan 1970b for overview) and the soma (see Perkins 1970 for overview) of stuttering to adequately diagnose and manage it. Our concern for the psychosocial adjustment problems of the young as well as older stutterer must not, of course, preclude our concern with these clients' speech behavior. It is real-

ized that after all is said and done, our index of clinical success with stutterers will be related to the amount of positive change we have brought about
in their speech behavior. If you will, the clinical proof of our success in
dealing with stuttering is in the pudding of the stutterer's speech behavior.
Unlike an individual afraid of snakes, who has successfully managed to avoid
snakes for years without anyone's noticing, our client's speech behavior is
there for the whole world to see and hear. Unless the stutterer essentially
avoids all speaking or happens to be a cave-dwelling hermit, sooner or later
he or she will have to speak. And if that stutterer has just gone through your
therapy program, every person he or she comes in contact with will shortly
know the relative success or failure of such therapy. Thus, our consideration
of stutterers' psychosocial concerns must take place in the context of our
simultaneous consideration of their speech behavior.

stutterers as people and as individuals

Our orientation to stuttering also includes the need to consider the
person who stutters as a person first and a stutterer second. The context of
the client's life cannot be ignored in our clinical dealings with that person.
Stutterers are people who have likes and dislikes, highs and lows, brothers
and sisters, dreams and schemes, just like everyone else. They share in the
same human condition that we all share. To remediate stutterers as if they
are isolates, with family, social, and other life issues in the background, is
not only inappropriate but also poor therapy. Speech-language pathologists
need to consider the context of the stutterer's life in order to see the
individual who stutters as a person, as a functioning individual interacting
on a number of levels with a number of people, and as a person, like you
and me, unique and without duplicate. Such a view helps us put into perspective the client's behavior during our remediation of that client. For
example, one teenage client we were treating was continually late or absent
from our early morning therapy appointments. This tardiness and absentee-
ism did not square with the client's in-therapy performance which indicated
fairly high levels of motivation. Knowing that the teenager's family was not
exactly wealthy, we began questioning him regarding whether he had an
alarm clock or any type of clock in his bedroom. He stated that he did not
have any such clock and that he relied on either the sun streaming through
his window or his mother to wake him up. Funds were generated to get this
young man an alarm clock, and we saw an end to his tardiness. What is the
point? Well, by assuming that the client was resisting our therapy, that he
really did not want help with his stuttering, we might have dismissed him
as just another unmotivated individual with a stuttering problem. However,
by realizing that there might be more to this client's life than just stuttering
(like serious monetary restrictions on family purchases), we were able to
resolve a relevant clinical issue. We wish that all our clinical problems were

so easy to solve! Keeping the perspective that the person who stutters is a person first, and a stutterer second, helps us to understand, if not to resolve, many such issues.

In considering stutterers as people, we must also consider each stutterer's individuality (Van Riper 1973). While there are commonalities among our clients, what may be appropriate in Sally's situation may not work with John. Gearing therapy procedures to the individual needs and abilities of various clients is not always easy, and not always possible. Nevertheless, we should at least recognize each client's individuality and not overly generalize. Procedures that make good sense to Mr. and Mrs. Brown for their little Joey may totally baffle and confuse Mr. and Mrs. Peterson in their dealings with their daughter Jane. Likewise, some clients will need the rationale and reason for each and every step of our clinical attempts to change their stuttering whereas others will simply want the procedure and we can forget the explanation. What takes one client one or two sessions to learn or understand may take another individual who stutters many sessions of intensive remediation. Reasons for these differences are not necessarily related to intelligence; such differences may relate to a stutterer's relative willingness to work at change, different levels of motivation, high degrees of emotionality surrounding the stuttering problem which make it difficult for the client to objectively deal with the problem, and so forth. In other words, while we must recognize certain commonalities among our clients who stutter, we must also recognize the range of individuals who surround, on both sides, such typicalness. Just as the fact that the average IQ is 100 does not mean that average people all have IQs equal to 100, so we find that all stutterers are not identical in terms of their problem and related concerns. To overgeneralize is to oversimplify.

rationales versus recipes

Last, but certainly not least, in our orientation to the problem of stuttering is our interest in understanding the reasons behind the method as well as the method itself. We want to try to understand why an advocated method is believed to work. We are not interested in simple recipes for clinical success that must dutifully be followed step by step.

If one does not know why a method is advocated, why it is thought to work, and how it might be adapted to each individual case, one may blindly follow one set of instructions in all therapy situations. Certainly therapeutic success of a particular method with stutterers is important; however, success, because of its highly elusive nature, is extremely difficult to determine. For example, what is meant by *success*? Who were the clients with whom the method was used? How long after therapy ended was stuttering behavior sampled? These and other questions can quickly put into perspective the many claims that this or that therapy procedure with stutterers results in 80 percent or 90 percent success (see Van Riper 1973, for a more complete overview of therapeutic success with stutterers). Even more important than the success issue is the ability to hand down the rationale for the therapy from one generation of professionals to another. Instead, too often, what is being handed down is procedure with no more justification for its working than the fact that it works, at least on occasion! This, I suppose, is fine as long as the procedure meets with some degree of clinical success. However, the day usually dawns when the procedure does not work with this or that client. Without knowing why the procedure was supposed to work in the first place, it is difficult for the clinician to adjust the procedure to meet the individual needs of the client.

Tightly structured programs for the remediation of stuttering may give clinicians the impression that they know what they are about, what they need to do, and how to do it. Such programs are many times suitable for certain stutterers or for certain aspects of certain stutterers; however, difficulties arise when exceptions to the rule or new information occurs that casts doubts on the prescribed program. We do not believe that we should confuse the confident manner of the cookbook-oriented clinician who works with stutterers with that clinician's expertise and ability to handle all clinical problems relative to stuttering. Such clinicians, in my experience, may reject or vigorously disagree with information or approaches that fall outside of the realm of their approach. Clinicians who seek and who learn the program seem to find it difficult to adjust to the clinical exception, new information, changing approaches. The *recipe approach,* particularly in view of our present state of the clinical art in stuttering, appears to hamper future growth in a clinician's ability to remediate stuttering.

problem solving versus *the program*

Problem solving (Carkhuff 1973), on the other hand, provides the speech-language pathologist with a general framework within which to ask meaningful questions and receive meaningful answers regarding stuttering (Williams 1968). Problem solving forces the clinician to take an active, leadership role in the diagnosis and management of stutterers. Problem solving encourages speech pathologists in the use of self-generated solutions to problems based on careful observations, testing, and evaluation. Problem solving eschews the rigid dogma inherent in *the program* and provides the clinician with a means to deal with the exceptions, new information, and new approaches. Problem solving approaches to stuttering provide insurance against the future because the future of our remediation of stuttering will certainly bring change. Even now, with the advent of such clinically applicable technology as microcomputers, clinical doors will open up for those speech-language pathologists flexible and broad enough to incorporate such technology into their therapy. We further believe that problem solving will not only allow us to keep an open mind to such new technology and/or developments but will also provide the tools with which to evaluate such new developments. Thus, for the short-run and for the "typical" client, *the technique* is somewhat attractive and certainly more of a security blanket for the clinician than a problem solving approach. For the future, however, where the emphasis will be on flexibility, growth, and expanded new clinical opportunities and technologies, a problem-solving strategy towards stuttering is far superior to a cookbook approach. Clinical techniques are not inherently evil; in the pages that follow we will examine and advocate a number of such techniques. Blind faith in a technique, however, to the exclusion of other approaches, is a pathway that seems to lead to minimal professional growth and development. Techniques are ill used when they are employed simply because they are all the clinician knows or is willing to learn.

So, where are we? We have spelled out some of our basic orientations to the remediation of stuttering. To briefly review, we must attempt to describe stuttering and related problems in as objective, behavioral terms as possible. We try to convey our orientation that speech-language pathologists can and are producing positive change in the speech and lives of individuals who stutter. This orientation, as stated earlier, is based on the realization that significant progress has been made in both our scientific understanding and our clinical treatment of stuttering. Such treatment needs to take into consideration the psychosocial as well as the speech-specific aspects of the problems of stuttering. The remediation of stuttering should involve the perspective that the stutterer is a person first and a stutterer second, and that as such a person, the client is unique and without duplicate. Problem-solving orientations to the remediation of stuttering are favored over cookbook approaches to the remediation of stuttering because problem solving allows the clinician to be more flexible, adaptive, and creative. Clinicians' ability to remediate stutterers will, of course, be importantly influenced by their ability to describe that which is called stuttering (see Robinson 1964; Van Riper 1971; Bloodstein 1975a overview). We would, therefore, like to present issues that I believe are necessary to consider when describing those events called stuttering.

O WHAT IS STUTTERING?: PERCEPTUAL CONSIDERATIONS

Listeners are most apt to perceive a speech disfluency as an instance of stuttering when a speaker produces a word that contains any one or a combination of the following: (1) a sound or syllable repetition, (2) a sound prolongation, or (3) an unusual pause between the sounds or syllables of that word. Of course, other types of speech disfluency are also sometimes associated with listener perceptions of stuttering (for example, repetitions of monosyllabic whole words like "I—I—I was here"). However, these other disfluency types, while not unimportant, are not the usual associates of listeners' perceptions of stuttering. Notice the phrase "listeners' perceptions of stuttering"; we need to be clear that perceptions of stuttering involve listener evaluations. We presently have no machines into which we can feed audiotapes of speech produced by suspected stutterers that can readily tell us (1) which sounds, syllables, words, phrases, or sentences contain stutterings and (2) whether the speaker who produced these speech events is a stutterer. We, the listener, must decide, after careful evaluation, whether we will consider a particular speech event as indicative of stuttering as well as who is and who is not a stutterer. And herein lies the problem: Judgments of stuttering involve perceptual evaluations and as when two or more people observe and report an event such as an auto crash, such judgments and evaluations are subjective, variable, and difficult to make.

Recognizing the variability and difficulty of making such perceptual evaluations need not preclude our developing a reasonably complete index of those events that are most apt to be perceived as stuttered. It is very difficult, if not impossible, to develop *absolute* definitions of what is and what is not stuttered and who is and who is not a stutterer (Bloodstein 1975a). However, it *is* possible to develop *relative* definitions of stuttering that capture the essentials of those speech units that listeners are apt to consider stutterings (Wingate 1964). The word *apt* is purposely used because this relative definition involves a statement of probability rather than one of certainty. For example, comics who attempt to imitate stutterers as part of their act are *apt* or *most likely* to select within-word rather than between-word disfluencies. The phrase *most likely* denotes an event that is relatively (probably) rather than absolutely (certainly) likely to occur. Once again, it is possible that listeners may perceive a particular between-word disfluency (for example, a revision) as stuttered and particular within-word disfluency (for example, a sound prolongation) as normally disfluent. It is possible but not as probable.

Besides those speech events which are most probably associated with listener perceptions of stuttering, listeners may also see and hear at least two other events associated with those events called stuttering: (1) (non)verbal reports of bodily movement and tension and (2) (non)verbal reports of psychosocial discomfort and concern (Bloodstein 1975a). These two events, along with the speech behavior itself, make up a behavioral composite which many speech-language pathologists have difficulty describing clearly and adequately. Indeed, the beginning speech-language pathologist may be so overwhelmed by these (non)verbal reports of bodily movement and tension and psychosocial discomfort and/or concern that he totally misses the client's actual speech behavior. Speech-language pathologists who remediate stuttering should be able to do what I call *parallel-process* (with all due apologies to my colleagues in speech science): simultaneously process or handle different types of information coming from different modalities. Remediating stuttering should not be undertaken by the clinician who cannot or will not simultaneously deal with different events, each of which has its own seriated time course and meaning.

Nonverbal and verbal reports of bodily movement and tension of the (non)speech musculature are commonly observed to be associated with stuttering (Brutten and Shoemaker 1967), particularly after the person has stuttered for some period of time. During instances of stuttering, the speech-language pathologist, or any other observant individual, may note the stutterer contracting and tensing muscles in and around the face, head, neck, and torso. Not as easily seen, but every bit as important, are the inappropriate contraction and tensing of muscles within the vocal tract (tongue, velar, mandibular, pharyngeal, and laryngeal areas). We may perceive these muscular contractions and tensings within the vocal tract as the stutterer using too much force to produce a particular speech event, such as an unusually long between- or within-word pause, and the like. These vocal tract behaviors may be associated with the instance of stuttering or they may be the peripheral reason that the person is actually stuttering. For example, if you were trying to sequentially touch your thumb tip to the tip of your index finger and then to your middle finger and so on to your baby finger, you might produce behavior that was either *associated* with your inability to move your thumb from one finger to the next (for example, stiffly locking your wrist to the left or the right) or that was actually the *reason* you could not move your thumb from one finger to the next (for example, pressing your thumb to your index fingers hard and not moving the thumbtip of the middle finger). In both cases, muscles would be seen to be contracted and tensed; however, in one case (wrist locking) muscle behavior would only be *associated with* the breakdown in forward thumb-to-finger movement and in the other (pressing thumb to index finger), muscle behavior would be the actual *reason for* the breakdown in forward thumb-to-finger movement. Thus, frequently, but not invariably, associated with stuttering are such behaviors as facial grimaces, tensing of neck muscles, rapid blinking and squeezing of muscles around the eyes, and so forth. Such behaviors may reflect the stutterer's belief that speech is difficult, that it takes work and force, and that it is something to be feared and dreaded.

Inappropriate bodily movement and tensing may also suggest that the stutterer is trying to cope with the stuttering itself. The head jerk to the right, neatly time-locked with the initiation of the articulatory contact of a feared sound or syllable, may indicate the stutterer's belief that this head jerking will "get the sound out." And as others have previously discussed (Williams 1971) if a little bit of movement and tensing helps, in this case head movement and neck muscle contracting, then a great deal more should really help! Unfortunately, these inappropriate behaviors occasionally appear to "work"! That is, by seemingly chance association with successful forward movement through a word, these behaviors appear to become reinforced in much the same way that the green shirt the pitcher wore on the day he pitched a no-hitter takes on special properties (see Skinner 1953 for discussion of superstitious behavior). Both the green shirt and the head jerking are seen by the pitcher and the stutterer, respectively, as being a help or as being essential to successful completion of the task at hand.

Along with these nonverbal and verbal reports of bodily movement and/or tension in (non)speech musculature, we may see and hear, from individuals who stutter, events indicative of psychological discomfort and concern. These reports (and they are generally, though not exclusively, verbal) may indicate fear, frustration, embarrassment, nervousness, anxiety, anger, and other such affective states. Basically, these reports indicate that during and/or in anticipation of moments of stuttering and of speech in general, the stutterer is in a state of emotional discomfort. In fact, the very act of stuttering (the repeating and prolonging of sounds) is taken by many to mean that the individual who produced them is tense, or nervous, or anxious. Disregarding these speech behaviors for the time being, what we are talking about here are such things as consistent aversion of eye contact with listeners that may be indicative of fear and anxiety and awareness of a problem. Even the body posture of the individual who stutters may appear different. We have noticed that when people have been stuttering for some time, their general body posture seems to become increasingly rigid or nonmovable when they speak, especially when they are about to stutter or are in the middle of an instance of stuttering. This observation, I hasten to add, is in need of empirical testing. Lack of eye contact, however, particularly in younger children, is generally a sign that all is not right regarding the children's feelings about themselves, their own speaking ability, and speaking in general (Ainsworth 1977). One thing we discuss, in later sections, are the feelings associated with some of the more common nonverbal and verbal reports of psychosocial discomfort. If we do not deal with these feelings, they may stand in the way of successful remediation.

It is interesting to note that certain aspects of both the nonverbal and verbal reports of bodily movement, tension and psychosocial concerns are of particular concern to the parents of the young stutterer. For example, parents often seem to show considerable concern regarding their child's facial grimacing, head jerking, and verbal reports of fear or embarrassment. However, these same parents, as well as other listeners and the stutterers themselves, may be less apt to show concern regarding sound prolongations than they are regarding sound-syllable repetitions. What we are trying to say is that there appear to be differential responses, on the part of the listener, to various aspects of a speaker's disfluent speech productions (for example, Williams and Kent 1958; Huffman and Perkins 1974). Not all aspects are judged as equally noxious; an individual listener may be particularly intolerant of a specific aspect of disfluent speaking behavior. We remember one mother who could listen all day to her son prolong sounds and not bat an eyelash; however, let that same son repeat the same sounds and the mother would respond with, "You know better than that," or "Stop that this instant."

Recapping, we consider as an instance of stuttering those speech events in which a word contains a sound-syllable repetition, a sound prolongation, or an inappropriate pause between sounds or syllables. Other events, as we have said, may also on occasion be considered as stuttering (for example, repetition of between-word interjections like "uh—uh—uh"); however, most speech behavior that is labelled by listeners as stuttering consists of within-word disfluencies. These within-word disruptions may be associated with one or both of the following: (1) nonverbal and verbal reports of bodily movement and tension in (non)speech musculature and/or (2) (non)verbal reports of psychosocial discomfort and concern. Within-word disfluencies are most apt to be perceived by listeners as stuttered (for example, Boehmler 1958; Williams and Kent 1958); this is a statement of relative rather than absolute certainty. We are still less than clear why listeners react in this way, but in later sections we present some speculation regarding such listener reactions. At this point, however, we shift our attention from perceptual considerations of stuttering to considerations of the development of the speech physiology associated with stuttering. The following description should not be considered as the *truth,* but rather as one possible means by which we can view the development of the abnormal speech physiology associated with stuttering. Although much has been learned in recent years regarding the disturbed speech physiology associated with stuttering, we are not in a position, at this writing, to pour such knowledge into concrete. Instead, we believe that we must be tolerant regarding the evolving state of the art and science of stuttering in this area and that we should be most willing to entertain *likely* rather than *certain* explanations.

O WHAT IS STUTTERING?: PHYSIOLOGICAL CONSIDERATIONS

We believe it safe to assume that the rather long duration sound prolongations of an adult stutterer with a severe stuttering problem did not develop overnight. Surely, when this adult stutterer was a child, his or her stuttering behavior was somewhat shorter in duration, probably less frequently exhibited, and possessed less audible manifestations of physiological tension than the adult form of the problem. However, what do we actually know about the beginning nature of stutterers' stuttering, particularly on the level of speech physiology? At present, the answer to the latter rhetorical question is very little despite the fact that many are currently engaged in the description of the actual physiological parameters of stutterers' (dis)fluent speech (for example, Conture, McCall, and Brewer 1977; Freeman and Ushijima 1978; Zimmerman 1980a, b; Shapiro 1980; Stromsta and Fibiger 1980). It would be particularly helpful to have information regarding the fluent speech of young children who eventually become stutterers to see whether there are aberrancies in their speech physiology even *prior* to the onset of these youngsters' stuttering. Such information would be most useful in clarifying the nature of the cause of stuttering as well as assist in early differential diagnosis of stuttering; however, the absence of this information should not preclude preliminary speculation regarding the physiological aspects of stuttering from its beginning through its later stage of development.

Table 1–1 presents just such speculation whereby the stutterer is viewed as moving through four interdependent stages, from beginning to end, in terms of physiological disruptions in fluent-disfluent speech. The first stage (*Alpha*) suggests that even in the fluent speech of young, potential stutterers we may find brief, nonperceptible (to listeners) aberrancies, for example, frequent inappropriate pauses between- and within-words, slightly longer than typical articulatory contact times or greater durations of voicing onset after consonantal release. It is unclear whether such *Alpha* behavior results from environmental or inherited (or both) factors, but recent findings of such disruptions, for example, Seebach and Caruso (1979), should begin to help in the early identification and positive therapeutic intervention of potential stutterers.

If we assume for the potential stutterer that *Alpha* behavior does not change with the child's maturation, we then posit that the next stage of behavior (*Beta*) would involve reiterative posturing of the speech production mechanism. These *Beta* behaviors would, in most cases, be apparent to most listeners and might be, in many children, the essential elements of what Johnson (1959) has termed *normal* nonfluency. It would seem that *Beta* behavior occurs when within-word pauses, articulatory contacts, or transitions occur for too long a duration and then the sound or syllable is reiterated.

Most children, we believe, develop out of this *Beta* behavior, but some children, for as yet unknown reasons, progress to *Gamma* stage. During *Gamma* stage, the young stutterer (we believe that using the term *stutterer* begins to become appropriate at the *Gamma* stage) demonstrates stabilized speech production whereby within-word pauses, contacts, or transitions are prolonged in time. In a sense, *Gamma* behavior is exaggerated (in terms of time and physiological effort and/or tension) *Alpha* behavior; that is, *Gamma* behavior differs in degree but not type from *Alpha* behavior. Interestingly, as will be mentioned later, our clients and their parents demonstrate much more concern about *Beta* behavior than they do *Gamma* behavior even though we and others (for example, Ainsworth 1977) believe that the stabi-

TABLE 1-1

The Possible Chronological Development of the Speech Physiology Associated with Stuttering

DEVELOPMENTAL STAGE	BEHAVIORAL DESCRIPTION	COMMENTS
Early Listed in order of Occurrence Later	(1) Alpha	(1) Brief, nonperceptible (to listener) *aberrancies* in speech production, for example, brief within-word pauses, laryngeal catches, or articulatory arrests at beginning of utterance or at transition between sounds and syllables	(1) *Alpha* resulting from one of three combinations of child and environment; Typical child speaking in unique environment or unique child speaking in typical environment or unique child speaking in unique environment
	(2) Beta	(2) Brief to lengthy repetitive speech productions used as compensatory and/or coping reactions to *Alpha*, for example, laryngeal adduction (inspiratory gesture and nostril flaring) alternating with adduction	(2) *Beta* results in sound-syllable repetitions; child "uses" *Beta* to adjust to, override, or release from *Alpha*
	(3) Gamma	(3) Brief to lengthy *stabilized*, relatively tense, speech production used as compensation or coping reactions to *Beta*, for example, fixed laryngeal adductory posture, labial contact, or lingual posturing	(3) *Gamma* results in sound prolongation; child uses this to minimize the highly variable, repetitive behavior of *Beta*; results in perceptually more acceptable behavior than *Beta* but still atypical end product
	(4) Delta	(4) Brief to lengthy *compensatory* speech productions used as coping reactions to *Gamma*, sometimes *Beta* and possibly in some instances, to *Alpha*; for example, pharyngeal muscle constriction, vocal fold lengthening (pitch rises), vocal fold shortening, where arytenoids approximate base of epiglottis (bearing down)	(4) *Delta* compensatory behavior may or may not have acoustic correlate, but probably does; one of more noticeable aspects of an instance of stuttering

13

lized, prolonged pauses, contacts, and transitions of this third stage are a definite step toward a worsening of the stuttering problem. The fourth, and final stage, *Delta,* is where the stutterer begins to produce a variety of speech (for example, inappropriate changes in vocal pitch) and nonspeech (for example, rapid aversion of eye contact and sideward movement of head) in apparent attempts to deal with *Gamma* behavior and the remnants of behavior left from the *Beta* and *Alpha* stages.

We are not trying to make definitive statements regarding these developmental stages of the physiological manifestations of stuttering but instead are saying that they seem to make sense to us in terms of our experience with stutterers and our own as well as others' research findings. The presence of *Alpha* behavior in the fluent speech of young stutterers is clearly discernable (although perhaps not to listeners), and we expect that the upcoming years will more definitively elaborate on such issues. We think it important that speech-language pathologists who work with stutterers begin to view fluency and stuttering along a continuum rather than as two completely different discrete events. That is, the slightly longer than normal stop phase of a young stutterer's /p/ in the fluent production of the word *popcorn* may only have to be maintained a bit longer, for example, 100 to 200 msec, and listeners begin to judge it as a silent sound prolongation or stuttering. Knowing the objective detail of these young stutterers' speech production should not cloud our view of these children as feeling, socially interacting individuals; however, neither should our consideration of these children's psychosocial activities obfuscate our detailed knowledge of their speech production.

We can and should consider both the physiological and psychological aspects of stuttering in our remediation efforts. Along these lines, we make three basic assumptions regarding the speech-language pathologist who remediates stuttering: (1) the best speech-language pathologist to work with stutterers is the individual who has the most information about stuttering and related matters; (2) this person must be able to clearly, logically, and sequentially organize this information for use in the remediation of stuttering; and (3) this person must be able to present that information in a way that makes sense to the stutterer (that the client can relate to) and that helps the stutterer. While the manner (presentation) of the speech-language pathologist comes under scrutiny of the client and other clinicians, we believe that our first assumption, the clinician's knowledge of stuttering, will dictate whether truly effective therapy will be carried out, particularly in the long run. And one significant part of that knowledge of stuttering is knowing something about the stutterers' speech physiology during both fluent and disfluent utterances. Let us now, however, turn our attention away from the behavior of stuttering towards the person who produces this behavior: the stutterer.

Do individuals automatically qualify as stutterers if they produce a within-word disfluency or two? The answer is most obviously no. Just as one swallow does not make a summer, neither does one instance of stuttering mean a person is a stutterer. Individuals who have just experienced one bout of alcoholic intoxification do not immediately seek out their local AA chapter; likewise, neither should a temporary period of within-word disfluencies mean that people should seek out therapy for stuttering. We become really concerned only when such within-word disfluencies persist over a sufficiently long period of time, when these disfluencies become predictable parts of their speech, and when these disfluencies come to be consistently associated with certain speech events and speaking situations. Before such persistence, predictability, and consistency of within-word disfluencies, we may observe and monitor individuals on a regular basis or, as others have suggested, provide parents with adequate information and appropriate counseling (Williams 1971; Ainsworth 1977). Such indirect therapy and parental counselling procedures will be dealt with later, but for now let us consider some of the more important facets in deciding who is and who is not a stutterer.

We mentioned previously that we become concerned and fairly sure that individuals are stutterers when within-word disfluencies are *predictable* parts of their speech, and when these disfluencies *persist* over sufficiently long periods of time, and when they are *consistently* associated with certain sounds-syllables, words, or speaking situations. We must remember, however, that the terms *persistent, predictable,* and *consistent,* for all their soundings of definitiveness and absoluteness, are still terms whose meaning is relative to the person who has stated them. We realize that we can go to extremes in stating that this or that is relative to its surrounds, but we have had many clinical experiences where one person's *persistent* is another person's *occasional.* Even in the presence of reports that a particular client is consistently stuttering, we should proceed with caution and avoid making a rush to judgment. I am not going to advocate a see-no-evil-hear-no-evil stance, but blasting onto the scene with plans for remediating stuttering on the basis of one person's report of chronic stuttering is not particularly appropriate.

My clinical experience indicates that speech fluency is one area of human behavior in which we have little tolerance for individual differences. We appear to accept the fact that some people can run and jump and climb farther, faster, and higher and at earlier ages than other people. We do not appear quite as tolerant, however, regarding differences among people in terms of speech fluency and speech and language behavior in general. Many individuals seem to be unwilling to accept the fact that some children go through periods of disfluency for longer periods than do other children or that some children go through these periods of disfluency at later or earlier periods than their peers do. For example, my son, when nearing his ninth birthday, went through a period of about two weeks in which he produced a fair number of whole-word repetitions and more than his normal amount of part-word repetitions. Other parents have reported to me increments in speech disfluency in the communication of their eight- to ten-year-old children. Are these instances of disfluency peculiar to this age range of children? Are they indicative of particular pressures we parents or the schools place on this age child? Are these disfluencies related to sudden spurts in vocabulary growth or language or cognitive development? Is this apparent discoordination of speech musculature (Perkins and others 1976; Perkins 1978) related to some as yet unknown neurological or physiological change peculiar to this age child? The answers to these questions are still vague, but we believe that judgments of the persistency, predictability, and consistency of speech disfluency and related events involves a person-by-person decision. We might like to use group norms (for example, more than 50 speech disfluencies per 100 words = stuttering) to assist us in establishing who is and who is not a stutterer; however, we still do not think the data are sufficient to provide us with good group norms. What is needed is more information, on a year-by-year or month-by-month basis, regarding the mean (plus range) number and type of disfluencies produced in children from say two to six years of age. Previous work in this area (for example, Davis 1939, 1940; Winitz 1961; Williams, Silverman, and Kools 1969; Yairi and Clifton 1972) is commendable, but the continued massive exposure to and influence of television and other medias on our children's language and cognitive development suggests that such work needs further updating and expanding.

People who are meaningfully considered to be stutterers are, therefore, generally consistent in terms of events that are associated with their instances of stuttering, persistent in their production of such disfluencies over a sufficiently long period of time, and predictable in that their speech can usually be described as containing disfluencies. Besides the disfluencies themselves, we might also expect consistent, persistent, and predictable verbal and nonverbal reports of bodily movement and tensing and psychosocial discomfort and concern. Also, some individuals consider themselves stutterers despite objective evidence to the contrary. Anyone who has evaluated and remediated the population of adult individuals referred to them for stuttering knows the difficulties of dealing with people who are objectively fluent but who subjectively feel they stutter and that they should be considered as stutterers (Douglass and Quarrington 1952; Prins 1974). Thus, besides that which we can hear and see (speech disfluencies, bodily movement, tension and psychosocial discomfort and/or concerns), we must also consider aspects of the individual's self-concept (for lack of a better phrase) that are not as easily viewed and heard. Individuals' consideration of themselves as stutterers cannot be ignored by the speech-language pathologist. Many times, careful observations of such fluent stutterers reveal a wide variety of subtle behaviors that the person is producing to get the sound out, or to avoid the word, or to circumlocute the situation, or sound, or word. These people, like their more disfluent peers, seem to universally complain that speech is a chore, that it is not automatic ("like everyone else"), and that they have to spend too much time thinking about *how* they are going to say something rather than *what* they are going to say. Other concerns exist for a number of these people; however, at this point let us state that the speech pathologist must be able to assess the nonobservable as well as the observable to determine who is and who is not a stutterer.

○ SOME PARTING THOUGHTS

In summary, individuals who *persistently, predictably,* and *consistently* produce within-word disfluencies within their verbal communications are likely candidates for being considered as stutterers. Their candidacy becomes even more likely if we observe, associated with these disfluencies, verbal and nonverbal reports of bodily movement, tension and psychosocial discomfort and concerns. Speech-language pathologists must recognize that such terms as *persistent, predictable,* and *consistent* are relative to both the observer and the observed. The mental, physiological, and chronological age of the client, in particular, needs to be considered in making judgments with regard to persistence, consistency, and predictability of stuttering. Finally, individuals' belief that they stutter and that they should be considered stutterers does not always square with the objective information available to the clinician. Truly ascertaining who is and who is not a stutterer is a complex decision based on many different considerations and, to some degree, relative to the particular clients, their age, and their internal feelings.

In later sections of this book, we deal in more detail with the making of this decision and the basis for making it. For now, let us realize the difficulties of such decision processes as well as that such decisions can and, in many instances, must be made for the benefit of the client and his or her relations. Although we can harm by rushing to judgment and remediating in situations where, given enough time, a problem might disappear, we also harm by not wanting to hurt the client. What is needed is an ability to know when to say an individual is truly a stutterer and in need of our services and the ability to know when to say an individual is truly not a stutterer, when the individual's disfluencies and related concerns, although perhaps present, are not sufficient or of a kind to warrant our services.

We would like to end this section by touching on an issue that was covered at the very beginning: our belief that speech pathologists can and are bringing about meaningful, positive change in the speech and related concerns of people who stutter. This belief is based on the fact that our profession has made tremendous strides over the last forty to fifty years in both our scientific understanding and our clinical management of the stuttering problem. Today, more than ever, we believe there is reason to think that our methods for helping stutterers, although far from perfect and in a stage of constant evolution, are routinely bringing about positive change in the speech and lives of individuals who stutter. I believe it more than appropriate to begin the following sections with hope and optimism that our services, as speech pathologists, can bring about significant change in the problem of stuttering.

SUMMARY

Stuttering most likely results from a complex interaction between the stutterer's environment (for example, parental standards for child behavior) and the abilities the stutterer brings to that environment (for example, gross/fine motor coordination). Listeners are most apt to perceive an instance of stuttering when they hear a within-word disruption, particularly a sound prolongation, within-word pause or sound, or syllable repetition. Generally, stuttering begins during childhood, and if the problem does not change by itself or through remediation, it continues to progressively develop with time through a series of stages which are still unclearly known but often speculated about.

Remediation of stuttering is helpful to many, particularly the younger clients, and in this author's opinion should involve modification of two factors: (1) the environment, for example, by means of parent counselling, and (2) speech-language behavior, for example, by changing inappropriate strategies for initiation of speech production. The author views individuals who stutter as people first and stutterers second. Within this viewpoint, the problem of stuttering has been defined and in subsequent chapters will be dealt with in terms of evaluation and remediation.

This book was not written to be taken as a cookbook for selecting this or that recipe to cure this or that aspect of stuttering. Instead, this book was written in an attempt to show and discuss the various things that need to be considered to understand, evaluate, and remediate stuttering. The orientation throughout is toward a problem-solving approach to stuttering that permits the speech-language pathologist to independently deal with the individual client according to the client's individualistic needs and concerns.

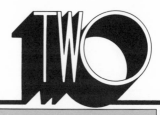

○ A FEW WORDS REGARDING THE EQUIPMENT USED IN EVALUATING STUTTERING

○ COMPONENTS OF THE STUTTERING EVALUATION

　　the intake form

　　the interview procedure

○ ASSESSING COMMUNICATIVE AND RE-LATED BEHAVIOR DURING THE STUT-TERING EVALUATION

　　fluency

　　hearing

　　voice

　　articulation

　　language

　　reading

　　intelligence

　　neuromuscular

　　psychological

○ WHO IS AND WHO IS NOT REFERRED FOR THERAPY

○ SUMMARY

Evaluation

Speech and language pathologists who remediate stuttering should have sufficient training in and experience with the evaluation of stuttering. It is, therefore, quite appropriate, before considering the remediation of stuttering, that we devote some time to considering its evaluation (for example, Williams 1974; Darley and Spriestersbach 1978). And as we see, the evaluation of stuttering, not unlike its remediation, presents a unique set of challenges and rewards.

The evaluation of stuttering requires the speech-language pathologist to consider what the client *is* as well as what the client *is not* saying and doing. It requires the clinician to consider the client's disfluent speech along with other related behaviors such as speech articulation, language, voice, reading, and so forth. The clinician may also need to consider the client's achievements and aspirations in terms of school and work, parental standards for child raising and behavior, parental concerns regarding spouses, and other such factors. All these considerations assist the speech-language pathologist in gaining perspective regarding the particular circumstances which surround each client's stuttering problem. For example, we gain this perspective when we consider that one stutterer may have limited intellectual and employment capabilities while another may have unlimited intellectual and employment capabilities. In evaluation, as in remediation, the examiner should remember that stuttering, in and of itself, does not encompass all of the client as a person nor the client's problems. Stuttering is but one of many components which go into making up individuals and their concerns.

Speech-language pathologists should also remember that their clients and associates will be evaluating them! And, as the saying goes, first impressions are important. It is therefore desirable that the client regards the clinician as being (1) a person concerned with both the client as a person and the client's problems; (2) a person who is nonjudgmental regarding both the client as a person and the client's problem; (3) a person who demonstrates a belief in the client's capacity for self-help; and (4) a person who demonstrates professional understanding and knowledge regarding the client's stuttering and related issues. Speech and language pathologists' evaluation of stutterers involves demonstrating to the client an understanding of stuttering while employing appropriate clinical affect and interpersonal skills. Shriberg and associates (1975) have detailed these professional, technical, and interpersonal skills, and Van Riper (1975) has discussed some of the clinical affect thought to be of relevance to successful clinical intervention. These professional and personal qualities of the clinician warrant consideration and study by any speech and language pathologist involved in the evaluation and remediation of stuttering and other communicative problems.

○ A FEW WORDS REGARDING THE EQUIPMENT USED IN EVALUATING STUTTERING

The ideal environment for evaluating stutterers should not possess auditory and visual stimuli which call *undue* attention to themselves. Distracting sights and sounds from outside and inside the evaluation room should be reasonably attenuated. While the evaluation room should not be overly cluttered, neither should it necessarily convey the sterility of a medical operating suite. For both the client as well as clinician the evaluation will take mental effort, concentration, and attention to detail, and the client may find it difficult to recall some of this detail from the backroads of his or her mind. We can assist the client with this task and reduce, as much as possible, distractions in the environment so that both the client and we can concentrate on the business at hand.

Although quite obvious, one very important piece of equipment in the evaluation of stuttering is the audio tape recorder and its associated microphone. Too often, we observe professionals who seem insensitive to the fact that high-quality acoustic tape recordings are crucial in the establishment of adequate behavioral indexes (baseline, before, or pretreatment measures) of stuttering. Most poor quality tape recordings of stutterings result from inappropriate microphone placement. Ideally, the recording surface of the microphone should be (1) placed perpendicular to the path or plane of the acoustic speech signal (for example, if the client is talking to a clinician across a table, the recording surface of the microphone should be pointed towards the ceiling or towards the wall to the client's immediate left or right) and (2) placed at a relatively constant distance from the client's lips and mouth. If both of these requirements for microphone placement are met, the next thing the clinician should insure is that the record gain of the tape recorder be set or regulated so that the recorded level of the speech is neither too low (soft) or high (loud); that is, the level of the recorded speech should be set so that the needle deflector on the VU meter is centering, during the recording, around the 0 mark. Not to put too fine a point on it, but if we seriously desire to achieve consistent, high-quality audio recordings of stutterers' speech behavior then we should not employ tape recorders that have glow tubes for VU meters, that lack VU meters, or that have built-in (nondetachable) microphones. Speech-language pathologists who desire audio tape recordings for the purposes of molecular and microscopic analysis of speech behavior (for example, vocalized versus nonvocalized pauses, voice quality associated with stutterings and so forth) are well advised to take the time necessary to set up and implement proper audio recording procedures. With practice, these recording procedures become second nature.

One last word regarding the environment of the stuttering evaluation concerns the clients' and their associates' right-to-know, or informed consent, regarding all of your clinical procedures and practices. In particular if the client and associates are to be observed, taped (either audio or audio-video), or otherwise scrutinized by yourself, your colleagues, or students-in-training, the client and associates should be so informed in as matter-of-fact a manner and tone as possible. Right from the beginning of the evaluation, providing the client an atmosphere of openness and honesty is important because the atmosphere we send out to clients many times indicates the atmosphere clients will send back to us. Telling a client that such observational procedures are routine and essential to help you help him is not only an honest but a wise policy. Surely, such openness may make some clients more visibly concerned when they know they are being observed and taped (they may ask many lengthy questions about the observational procedure and the use to which the observed information will be put as well as who is doing the observing), but it is clearly the right of the client to know such matters. After all, it is more than likely that this is the way you would want to be dealt with if you were in your client's shoes.

○ COMPONENTS OF THE STUTTERING EVALUATION

Disregarding, for the moment, the age of the client you will evaluate, the *ideal* evaluation of stuttering should include the following components: (1) An intake form, filled out in advance of the evaluation by the client and/or parent(s), teacher, doctor, and so on, providing identification plus basic information regarding history of the problem and related matters; (2) An interview with the client and, if available, associates, regarding history, current and possible future status of the problem plus motivation, need and desire for clinical services; and (3) standardized and nonstandardized assessment of communicative and related skills. None of these three components takes ascendence during the evaluation, but certainly, in my experience, those aspects of the evaluation which involve the clinician's interviewing skills are those parts which seem the most difficult to master.

the intake form

The first component, an intake form, should ideally have been completed in advance of the evaluation, and it should include information regarding identification of client and associates as well as general information regarding history of problem and related matters. It is important to obtain complete and accurate identification information: addresses, zip codes, telephone numbers (home and office), complete birthdate and date of evaluation (day, month, and year), present occupation, education and so forth. This type of information is all too often neglected, missing, or inaccurate; however, it often serves as the basis for the clinician's first remarks to the client. Identification information is also invaluable for follow-ups after the evaluation, in making referrals, planning remediation, and so forth. Furthermore, the client's or parents', in case of the child, taking the time in advance to complete such forms suggests that the client is at least willing to expend some effort in self-help. Consequently, when an evaluation begins without the client's having completed or only partially completing the form, we ask ourselves the following question: If this client is not willing and able to find the time to expend the effort to fill out such forms, how willing and able will he or she be to put the necessary time and effort into speech therapy?

the interview procedure

The second component of the stuttering evaluation consists of the clinician questioning the client and associates regarding the *who, what, where, when,* and *why* of the stuttering problem (see Appendix A for examples of such questions). The clinician's questions should be asked in as open-ended a form as possible and if the client does not provide an appropriate response, asked again, albeit in another form. If the clinician wants black and white, yes and no responses from the client, then questions can be structured accordingly ("Are you a boy?"). However, if the clinician wants more expansive, more informative responses (which is generally the case), then he or she can ask questions which lead the client to respond in a like fashion ("Why do you think you stutter?").

The clinician must also follow up on many of the client's responses to questions with further questions; however, knowing when and how to follow up is a most difficult skill to learn in becoming a successful interviewer. For an actual example of follow-up, consider the situation where we suspected a father of having unreasonably high standards for his daughter's verbal communication. The father said, in an extremely fluent, articulate fashion, that he had always had to sell himself through verbal communication. Following up on this comment, we asked the father about his boyhood and that of his relatives, and he said that both he and his father had been champion debaters in school and had won many individual as well as team honors. We then asked him to tell us about his debating experience, and the father stated that he had hoped the family tradition of debating would be carried on by his daughter and that he had been helping her learn to develop the necessary communication skills. Unfortunately, at that time his daughter was but eight years of age and not exactly what we would consider an oral-laryngeal athlete! This information, developed from our follow-up questions, together with other observations, lead us to suspect that the father had somewhat unreasonable standards for his daughter's verbal communication. It is not that the father was not going to tell us about his debating days (although sometimes this is the case); it is just that he did not think it too relevant. And, perhaps, such information might not be too relevant; however, we cannot consider the relevance of anything unless we have the thing to consider in the first place! Follow-up to client's responses, we have found, often provides the things we need to consider. We should not, we hasten to add, use follow-up as free license to snoop and poke through all our stuttering client's personal dirty laundry. However, if the clinician thinks the information necessary to understand and thus help the client, then the information is worthy of the clinician's attempts to retrieve it.

Besides follow-up, we need to consider the general nature of questions that we ask during the interview part of the stuttering evaluation. At least three types of questions are asked by the speech pathologist during the evaluation of stutterers:

1. A question clinicians ask themselves about the client which leads them to test the client to find the answer(s), for example, "Is this client more or less fluent when he or she reads or speaks?"

2. A question clinicians directly ask the client, his or her parents, or associates, for example, "Why do you want, at this point, to receive speech therapy?"

3. A question clinicians ask themselves about the client which requires inferences to find the answer(s), for example, "What is the source of this person's desire to receive speech therapy (parental, peer, spouse, or employment pressure)?"

The first type of question (questions leading to testing) is quite familiar to most clinicians: Is the client more fluent when reading than when speaking? On the average, how many of the client's words per 100 words spoken are stuttered? What is the client's most frequently produced disfluency type? Are the client's hearing, articulation, and language skills within normal limits? Can we get clues from the client's voice quality that indicate how the larynx is operating during stuttering? Are the client's intellectual and reading skills of a nature to allow this person to derive sufficient benefit from remediation at this point in his or her life? These and other questions like them form the essence of what a speech pathologist will need and want to ask of the client who is suspected or known to stutter.

The second type of question (questions directly asked of the client and associates) is most likely to be asked during an interview with the client, parents, or associates: How would you describe to me your or your child's stuttering speech behavior? Would you please show or demonstrate for me how you or your child stutter? What is your theory of why you or your child stutter? Did your stuttering (or your child's stuttering) begin with a prolonging or repeating of sounds and syllables? What types of therapy have you or your child previously received? Why did such therapies help or not help you or your child? What are your or your child's general strengths or weaknesses? A listing of questions can be found in Appendix A; hopefully this list will serve as a guide to you in the development and implementation of your own interview procedure. By no means, however, should such a listing preclude or restrict you from developing different and additional questions to be used for your own interview procedure.

The third type of question (questions answered by inference and guesstimation) is also important in the evaluation of stutterers. Interestingly, clinicians frequently do not seem to even realize that they are asking or need to ask such questions. The speech and language pathologist must develop some ability to judge but not be judgmental of people and their actions. The clinician must be able to judge the client in terms of whether the client has sufficient skills or has the potential for developing skills to make the necessary changes in speech and related behavior. To arrive at such judgments, clinicians will find themselves asking themselves the following types of questions: Is this person capable of expending the necessary mental and physical effort and time to change behavior? What is the source of the motivation and desire for therapy (Prins 1974; Starbuck 1974)? Why is this person seeking services? How reliable, honest, and straightforward is this client in his or her responses to me? Does this person really appear to understand what I am saying and asking? Is this client assuming a *cure me* role (passive consumer), or is he or she assuming a *self-effort with guidance* role (active producer)? Are these parents setting reasonable standards for child behavior and child raising?

Of course, these questions are not asked independently of one another; they obviously dovetail and are at times redundant in terms of the information they provide. Redundancy, however, is not necessarily a bad thing in evaluation since it provides a means for checking on the consistency and stability of the client's statements and behavior. The point is that the type of question the speech-language pathologist asks is not restricted to this or that section of the evaluation. In fact, the answer to one type of question may partly or completely answer another type of question. Let us now consider the specific *wh* questions that we directly ask clients and their associates during the interview.

Who. The who of the stuttering evaluation relates as much to the person(s) who considers the client as a stutterer as it does to the client himself. Johnson's (1961) ear-of-the-listener idea still has relevance if from no other standpoint than discovering the client's most critical listener(s). If the client is an adult, the who is often shrouded in the fog of the past events;

however, with the child, the who is more easily discernible as well as more immediately involved. Even for adult stutterers, it is important to discern who has considered and who does consider them a stutterer and the nature of their relations. It is not uncommon for the adult stutterer, particularly one who is quite fluent, to be considered a fluent speaker by most if not all of his or her listeners (Prins 1974). In later chapters, we discuss speaker problems that do not appear as problems to listeners, but because the speaker considers them problems, they become so!

What. The what of the stuttering evaluation basically involves having the client and associates describe what behaviors they are calling stuttering. This, unfortunately, is not as easy as it appears. First, clients, when asked to show you what they do that they call stuttering, will typically respond with, "It's hard to do . . . I can't do it on command . . . I'd rather not . . . I can't imitate it . . . It won't sound like real stuttering." Many times clients describe *in words* rather than *showing you* that which they do which they call stuttering. It is important during the initial evaluation for clients to actually *show you* (demonstrate for you) what they do that they consider stuttering. We also like to see if the client's associates can demonstrate or show you that which they consider stuttering. Both the client's and associates' *ability* to show you and their relative *willingness* to do so is quite instructive with regard to their objectivity, awareness, and knowledge of the speech problem. Secondly, the client may be calling some behaviors stuttering which are not stuttering. Although it seems strange, we have clients call something a stuttering problem when their problem was really a concern with voice, misarticulation, expressive-receptive language, dialectical articulation-language usage, neuropathologies of speech, hearing, or even vision! It is, therefore, imperative to sort out the *real* from the *imposter* stuttering! Third, it is not uncommon for a client to have more than one speech problem; for example, we just evaluated a boy (by means of perception, accelerometry [Stevens, Kalikow, and Willermain 1979], and videofluoroscopy [Skolnick and McCall 1972]) who has, besides his stuttering, a slight degree of velopharyngeal incompetence. This problem seems to contribute to his slight, but consistently inappropriate, nasal voice quality which is present in both the fluent and disfluent portions of his speech. Detailed observation indicates that he does not have either an apparent or submucosal cleft, but that the lateral aspects of his pharyngeal walls do not make quite enough contact or closure with the sides of the velum. Which came first: the stuttering or the nasal voice quality? Which causes which: the stuttering as reaction to the nasal voice quality or vice versa? Does the nasal voice problem suggest a residual from a previous neuropathology, or is it a case of faulty learning? Is there any relation between the stuttering and the nasal voice quality? Of course, we have no definitive answers to these questions, but we do know that a thorough evaluation of stuttering requires that we ask such questions.

Where. The where is closely related to the when of stuttering except that it specifically relates to the situations and listeners associated with instances in which stuttering is more or less apt to occur. A situational hierarchy (Brutten and Shoemaker 1967) elucidates for the clinician the association between various situations and the client's stuttering. Such a hierarchy also helps the clinician discern how clear and objective the client is regarding situations and listeners which relate to the client's stuttering. Our clinical observations suggest that clients who provide descriptive, detailed situational hierarchies have a better prognosis than those who cannot or who experience great difficulty in doing so.

When. The when of the stuttering evaluation refers not only to when the instance of stuttering occurs but also to when the onset of stuttering began. How old was the child and how long has the child been exhibiting this behavior? In Appendix B we present a case example of a child and his mother whom we were able to evaluate very shortly after the onset of the problem. In this case, we were able to describe the when of the onset of the stuttering with much more detail than is typically the case. The other when ("when do instances of stuttering occur") is most apt to be reacted to by such statements as, "I don't know, they just occur any old time . . . Somedays I'm good and somedays I'm bad . . . There just doesn't seem to be any rhyme or reason . . . Johnny goes for days and is fluent and then for several weeks he stutters his head off." Truly, for both the client and clinician, this apparently random waxing and waning, this apparent episodic or cyclic variation of stuttering is a most perplexing and discouraging aspect of stuttering (Robinson 1964). One of the first tasks that the clinician must undertake in evaluation and subsequent therapy is to circumscribe the when of the stuttering and assist the client (and associates) in seeing the regularity and consistency of the relations between events and stuttering. As long as the client reacts to the problem in a passive, "it's happening to me" fashion (Williams 1957), the client will have difficulty coming to grips with and changing behavior. The when and where of instances of stuttering, at least for the advanced stutterer, can become a means by which the clinician can begin to help clients see the relation between their speech, themselves, and their speaking environment.

Why. It is an ambitious undertaking, to say the least, to try to answer the question of why a person stutters. In a sense, when we ask why one person stutters, we are asking why all people stutter. Our answer to such questions will be dictated, in large degree, by our theory or those of others of why people stutter. Conversely, some clinicians may believe that theories of why stutterers stutter are of little therapeutic import. Such clinicians may believe that because we can never really know why a person stutters that it is meaningless to ask and that all one needs to know are what behaviors are in error and what behaviors one wants the client to produce. However, the

truth undoubtedly lies somewhere between, on the one hand, antitheoretical behavioristic tenets and on the other, elaborate, but empirically nontest-
able theory (see Guitar and Peters 1980 for some comparison and
amalgamation of these two points of view). It is obvious some form of theory
underlies the thinking of even the antitheoretical behaviorists: It is their
theory that behavior is of relevance and that behavior should be discussed
and dealt with in behavioral terms. Conversely, theory that leads nowhere,
which is fundamentally unprovable, is of small immediate assistance, albeit
in the long run it may lead to important new discoveries. Bloodstein (1975a)
makes a good statement in this regard, "A theory may be poor, not primarily
because it is untrue, but because it is logically incapable of verification as
stated".[1] Nevertheless, it is instructive to ask the client and his or her
associates what their theories of stuttering are to see what they believe
started or caused the stuttering problem. It is also instructive to try to
determine, from the evaluator's perspective, why a person continues to
stutter. Many times such questioning leads the evaluator to areas that contribute to or maintain, if not cause, the problem of stuttering. So, although
it is still a bit pretentious to claim that we know what causes stuttering
(Wingate 1964), it is still of clinicial benefit to keep asking the question.

With the intake form in hand and the results of the interview obtained,
the speech-language pathologist then may turn to the third component of
the evaluation: the actual assessment of communicative and related behavior. If the interview places a premium on appropriate questions and adequate follow-up, the actual assessment of communicative and related
behavior places a premium on careful observations. The idea that behavior
can be within normal limits but different from the mean is a concept which
is crucial to master and appreciate if a speech pathologist is to evaluate
fluency and related events.

○ ASSESSING COMMUNICATIVE AND RELATED BEHAVIOR
DURING THE STUTTERING EVALUATION

fluency

Assessing stuttered speech requires that the clinician consider some
or all of the following: (1) Type of disfluency (for example, part-word
repetition versus revisions); (2) Mean and range of frequency of each disfluency type with particular reference to which type is most and which type is
least frequent (for example, 4 part-word repetitions per 100 words spoken

[1]O. Bloodstein, *A Handbook on Stuttering* (Chicago: National Easter Seal Society for
Crippled Children and Adults, 1975), p. 64. Reprinted by permission of the author
and publisher.

versus 0.5 revisions per 100 words spoken); (3) Mean and range of frequency of total disfluency per 100 words spoken plus percentage of this total
contributed by each disfluency type; (4) The mean and range of duration of
within-word disfluencies (a digital stopwatch is most useful for recording
this temporal measure); (5) Percent of adaptation of stuttering frequency
across successive readings or speaking of identical material; (6) Consistency
of instances of stuttering and aspects of speech and language more or less
associated with these instances. Other factors, such as vocal quality associated with stutterings, reading and speaking rate, and so forth, may also be
considered; however, from the preceding six we can obtain the essentials for
defining and describing instances of stuttering and the nature and degree
of the stuttering problem.

These essentials can be abbreviated into the following five considerations: (1) What is the nature, frequency, and consistency of the behavior
called stuttering? (2) Is the disfluency primarily within-word as opposed to
between-word in nature? (3) What percent of the client's total disfluencies
are within-word? (4) Is the total frequency of disfluency within normal limits
for the age and communicative skill of the client? (5) Is the frequency of
within-word disfluency outside of normal limits for the age and communicative skill of the client? Although we still have less than adequate norms for
speech fluency, our experience suggests that individuals with much more
than an average of about two to three *within-word* disfluencies per 100 words
spoken (averaged across various types and complexities of speaking situations) have some degree of fluency problem (this frequency of within-word
disfluencies does not mean, however, that the individual is a stutterer). The
younger the client, of course, the less reliable any such absolute percentages
become because of the still-developing nature of the young child's communicative skills. The consistency of disfluency can be judged on an informal
as well as the more formal basis described by Johnson and associates (1963).
Although we are still less than clear regarding the exact clinical significance
of consistency of disfluency, I use this information as one more piece of data
regarding the relative habituation and association of the stuttering with
particular stimuli. Knowing the nature of the various types of stimuli, which
have been well documented elsewhere (see, Bloodstein 1975a, pp. 201–
202), allows the clinician to show the client that stuttering is associated with
specific, predictable events and situations, that stuttering has some degree
of lawfulness—that it is not a random event behaving helter-skelter like so
many kernels of corn popping in a popcorn popper.

As the problem of stuttering develops, the actual instances of disfluency
are associated with a wide variety of nonspeech behaviors such as eye blinking, facial grimaces, nostril flaring, head jerking and nodding, and other
bodily movements. Much has been said regarding these overt-covert bodily
movements and behaviors (see, Bloodstein 1975, pp. 10–16) and whether
they are used to avoid (occur prior to) or escape (occur during) an instance

of stuttering. However, many stutterers during speech, particularly during stutterings, also exhibit a *lack* of movement or what I call a bodily rigidity. This bodily rigidity is not to be confused with body rigidity resulting from neuropathology (see Darley, Aronson, and Brown 1975); the rigidity appears self-imposed or produced. The stutterer appears to stiffen the torso and/or arms and legs into a fixed or relatively nonmobile posture. The usual amount of bodily movement and gesture observed during the speech of fluent speakers appears missing during the speech of stutterers. Stutterers' bodily posture during speech conveys the message that these people (the stutterers) are not relaxed, that they are working at something that takes great effort and that they are anxious and concerned regarding their speech and themselves. Stutterers may be trying to stabilize their entire bodily posture in attempts at producing the sound, syllable, or word. Perhaps, like an individual with a shaking hand who tenses his or her hand, wrist, forearm, and shoulder to stop the hand from shaking, stutterers may tense the entire body to minimize the "shaking" in their speech or at least to help them cope with speaking. Of course, such bodily tensing is counterproductive to fluent speech in which the musculature must exhibit neither too much nor too little tonus. To our way of thinking, *absence* of normal bodily movement and gesture during speech is as characteristic of stuttering as is *presence* of abnormal bodily movement (for example, head jerks, facial grimaces, and so forth).

hearing

Besides the disfluencies themselves and their ancillary (non)speech associates, the speech pathologist must consider other aspects of communication: hearing, voice, articulation, and language. If at all possible a pure tone screening (air and bone) and speech discrimination testing should be done. It is not uncommon for stutterers to exhibit some history or presence of middle-ear concern: frequent earaches, ear-drum rupture, persistent fluid in the ear, surgically inserted pressure-equalizing tubes, and so forth. Such problems need to be considered because they may mean that the child who stutters, who also has chronic middle-ear problems, is not always going to have the best auditory sensitivity-discrimination. It may also mean that the child may be tired and more prone to fatigue as a result of frequent middle-ear infections (and associated upper respiratory infections) in addition to the medication used to remediate such problems or the excessive postnasal secretion brought about by a client's allergy.

voice

Voice problems (see Boone 1977 for overview of various types of voice problems and therapies for same) as well as articulation and language

TABLE 2-1

Voice Onset Time (VOT) during *Fluency* of Children and Adults who Stutter

The mean and standard deviation (SD) of young stutterers' (N = 8) and normally fluent speakers' (N = 8) VOT during *fluency* are given (in msec) for three voiced (/b d g/) and three voiceless (/p t k/) stop plosive consonants. Although greater absolute differences exist between talker groups for voiceless than for voiced stops, there are also greater absolute VOT values for voiceless than for voiced stops. Thus, there is more opportunity for greater absolute differences for voiceless than voiced stops because we are dealing with larger values of VOT for the voiceless than for the voiced stops. For sake of comparison, VOT data is provided for adult stutterers and normally fluent speakers during *fluency*

| | CHILDREN[1] | | | | ADULTS[2] | | | | ADULTS[3] | |
| | Normally Fluent (N = 8) | | Stutterer (N = 8) | | Normally Fluent (N = 5) | | Stutterer (N = 5) | | Normally Fluent (N = 3) | |
Sound	Mean	SD	Mean	SD	Mean	SD	Mean	SD	Mean	Range
/b/	14.9	2.7	20.1	5.5	13.5	5.0	27.8	8.5	11	6–14
/d/	17.4	3.5	25.2	4.9	23.2	9.7	33.4	11.8	17	11–23
/g/	29.0	6.6	32.0	9.2	32.7	8.7	41.8	5.2	27	19–36
/p/	64.7	18.3	92.0	16.0	52.3	8.7	68.0	11.1	47	42–50
/t/	65.7	14.9	96.6	18.1	69.4	7.8	77.2	15.2	65	53–77
/k/	68.7	13.6	96.2	16.1	73.9	9.3	79.8	14.6	70	66–74

[1] Seebach and Caruso (1979)

[2] Metz, Conture & Caruso (1979)

[3] Klatt, "Voice Onset Time, Frication and Aspiration in Word-Initial Consonant Clusters," *Journal of Speech Hearing Research*, 18, (1975), 686–706. Reprinted by permission of the author and publisher.

problems have every bit as much right to occur in stutterers as they do in the normal population. We have *little* documented evidence regarding stutterers' typical voice problems, for example, vocal nodules resulting from hyperfunctional vocal use (see Freeman 1979 for overview of this area). However, laryngeal disturbances are associated with actual instances of stuttering (Conture, McCall, and Brewer 1977; Freeman and Ushijima 1978), and there is some evidence that abnormal laryngeal behavior is also associated with stutterers' fluent speech (Adams and Hayden 1976; Hillman and Gilbert 1977; Cross and Luper 1979; Metz, Conture, and Caruso 1979; Seebach and Caruso 1979). Table 2–1 depicts such differences between the fluency of normally fluent and stuttering youngsters in terms of voice onset time measures; Table 2–1 also provides comparable information for the fluent productions of normally fluent adults and stutterers. The precise meaning of these relatively subtle differences in laryngeal behavior between the fluent speech of stutterers and normally fluent speakers is still less than clear (see Metz, Conture, and Caruso 1979), but it does seem that we, as speech-language pathologists, should know of the existence of such differences and support further exploration into their exact nature and possible underlying cause(s).

Clinically, we have observed individual children and adult stutterers who exhibit little or no pitch variability during speech, or whose modal pitch appears lower than it should be, or whose vocal quality is not especially good. We hasten to add, however, that we have not observed in either a frequent or consistent manner the fact that stutterers possess any *one* particular voice problem, for example, hoarseness, harshness, and so forth. Clearly, a stutterer may exhibit a voice problem, but it is our experience that articulation and language problems are just as, if not more, frequently associated with stuttering than voice problems and that stutterers' speech articulation and language concerns warrant our attention.

articulation

If stutterers misarticulate (see McDonald 1964; Shriberg and Kwiatkowski 1980 for examples of various means of assessing speech sound production), they are most apt, like their normally fluent peers, to misarticulate fricatives, particularly /s/, and some glides, like /r/ and /l/. For the adult stutterer, these speech misarticulations seem, for the most part, to be slight and of no serious consequence. With the younger stutterer, however, particularly the one who appears to be slow and/or deviant in the development of speech and language, speech misarticulations are of no small concern. I have seen youngsters brought in too early for speech therapy for their articulation problem with the result that all the children really learn is what sounds are their *problem sounds* and that they have to work to correctly produce these sounds. This form of speech therapy is even more detrimental when its major focus is phonetic placement (that is, the clinician stresses the correct articulatory placement for a particular sound) (Winitz 1969). This phonetic placement procedure, in our experience, is not only counterproductive to facilitating fluency but has the potential for exacerbating the stuttering problem. One notable exception, however, is the obvious need for some form of articulation therapy when the child exhibits marked speech unintelligibility and concern over his or her inability to orally communicate.

Much more needs to be explored in this area, but for now we should be cautious when during the course of an evaluation a young stutterer also exhibits noticeable speech misarticulations.* It is better for the child to receive no speech therapy than a therapy that exaggerates and stresses overarticulation and physically tense speech articulatory musculature and posturing. Any therapy or procedure is contraindicated that develops within the young child who stutters the idea that speech is hard, that speech takes work and effort, and that speech is something that requires caution. Many of these problems can be alleviated with patience on the part of the clinician and counselling of the parents; I believe it is most prudent to take a wait-and-see attitude.

---

*Such misarticulation may even be appropriate for the child's chronological age or developmental level of achievement.

language

Language difficulties can also accompany stuttering; however, the frequency and nature of such language concerns with stutterers is still unclear. It does seem with the occasional client, particularly children, that the length and complexity of their language structures are less than appropriate for their age (see Table 2–2). Other children seem to be less than adequate for their age in sequentially relating a story or event to a listener. Other children seem to persist in a continuing monologue to the extreme frustration and boredom of their listeners. Whatever the case, both nonstandardized and standardized assessments of language are in order particularly with stuttering clients referred to you who are from two to ten years of age. We have taken the approach that when children's language problems are more evident and detrimental than their fluency problem, these children should receive remediation and stimulation of language behavior. When both language and fluency are of equal concern, one has a more difficult choice; both aspects of communication may need simultaneous remediation. Of the three major communication problems (language, articulation and voice) that may be associated with stuttering, I have found that language stimulation and remediation can be most facilitative and least disruptive to an ongoing program of fluency therapy.

reading

Other skills like reading and academic subjects can have both direct and indirect relation to stuttering. Obviously, if a child is having oral reading difficulties, these difficulties may contribute to his stuttering during reading. Although we reported that young stutterers' reading ability is not significantly different from that of normally fluent speakers (Conture and Van Naerssen 1977), any one particular stutterer may have a reading concern that warrants attention from a reading specialist before speech therapy can begin. If the client has a reading difficulty, it makes for difficulty in speech therapy if reading material is used as a means of working on speech behavior. Academic problems can be a problem in speech therapy if the child is having so much trouble with school subjects that he or she feels discouraged or lacking in confidence and regards any new situation like speech therapy sessions as a threat. Further, a child struggling with school work, particularly if that child is still doing poorly, is a child who is tired at the end of the school day. Such fatigue needs to be taken into consideration by a speech pathologist planning therapy for that child.

intelligence

Intelligence, to the extent that we can adequately measure such an elusive commodity, is a factor in all learning experiences, and therapy with

TABLE 2-2

Typical Data Obtained from Young Children Who Stutter (N = 8)

Note that the male subject who is 5 years 6 months has questionable articulatory-language-vocabulary skills in addition to stuttering; however, other clients, for example, the 4 year 6 month male, have more adequate skills in these areas. Data suggest need for differential diagnosis (see Gregory 1973) and consideration of each client's individual needs and abilities.

EIGHT CHILDREN WHO STUTTER

Sex	Age at Time of Test		Number of Within-Word Disfluencies per 100 Words		Duration of Disfluencies		Articulatory Errors			Mean Length of Utterance	Inconsistent or Missing Grammatical Morphemes	PPVT	SP
	Years	Months	Mean	Range	Mean	Range	Dis	Sub	Omit				
Male	3	5	12	0–40	0.87	ERT–1.46	1	9	0	5.34	0	–N	14/50
Male	3	11	38	22–43	1.10	ERT–1.50	4	8	1	4.4	0	N	40/50
Male	4	6	6	5–8	0.61	ERT–1.09	0	4	1	5.2	2	N	24/50
Male	5	6	14	0–25	0.82	ERT–1.50	1	1	1	4.8	4	–N	17/50
Male	5	10	8	3–12	0.56	ERT–1.27	0	0	0	8.2	0	N	16/50
Male	5	8	15	5–40	1.00	0.42–2.00	0	10	2	4.8	1	N	41/50
Male	6	3	7	4–9	0.35	ERT–0.53	0	0	0	6.5	0	N	18/50
Male	8	2	7	0–20	0.80	0.3 –1.6	2	7	3	5.1	5	–N	5/50

ERT = Examiner's Reaction Time

Dis = Distortion

Sub = Substitution

Omit = Omission

PPVT = Peabody Picture Vocabulary Test

N = Within Normal Limits (–N = Below normal limits)

SP = Stocker Probe Test (50 items, the more the child stutters the higher the score) stutterers is no exception. We have used psychometric test findings reported to us by psychologists as well as scores from such tests as the Quick test (Ammons and Ammons 1962) to get some general idea regarding the client's intellectual functioning. It should come as no surprise that we have found that more intelligent clients seem to move through therapy at a more rapid pace and seem to make more lasting changes. However, we are still uncertain regarding the relation between stutterers' intelligence and their therapeutic progress; we need to more systematically investigate this relationship (see Sheehan 1970 for overview). Certainly, we have never excluded a subject from consideration simply on the basis of intelligence; instead we try to tailor all our therapy procedures to meet the needs of the individual client.

neuromuscular

Neuromuscular skills in nonspeech and speech tasks warrant some discussion. It is not uncommon for a client to demonstrate marginal skills in certain fine and/or gross motor tasks, particularly tasks that require rapid, sequential, and coordinated use of musculature (for example, rapidly and sequentially touching tip of thumb to each finger tip). Some stutterers will exhibit difficulty touching their tongue tip to either the middle of their upper lip or the middle of their chin, just below their lower lip. Some stutterers may show awkwardness in rapidly moving their tongue from side to side; however, none of these skills, even for the normally fluent population, have been adequately shown to relate to speech difficulties (see Hardy 1970, 1978). Alternate and sequential motion rate tasks (Darley, Aronson, and Brown 1975), however, do show a relationship to stuttering problems. A number of stutterers, particularly those who seem to have a more severe and habituated problem, will stutter on the first mono-, bi-, or tri-syllable produced in either an alternate or sequential motion rate task. This stuttering usually takes the form of an audible or silent prolongation of the syllable-initial sound of the first syllable in the string, after which they generally produce the remaining syllables in a fluent manner. Excluding this initial stuttering, the fluent syllables are generally produced at a rate that is within normal limits. Stuttering during alternate and sequential motor tasks indicates a very habituated problem as well as a poor prognosis.

psychological

Psychological factors to consider during the stuttering evaluation basically involve three aspects: (1) motivation for seeking services; (2) psychological aspects that may hinder or facilitate therapeutic progress; and (3) psychological considerations that warrant referral to other professionals, for example, a clinical psychologist or a psychiatrist. While there can be no denial that psychological factors play a part in stuttering, neither our experience nor our research supports the claim that such factors predominate (see Sheehan 1970a). Most of the psychosocial aspects that we see in the problem of stuttering appear to be "normal reactions to abnormal situations, environments, or people." It is hard, if not impossible, to remain calm when speaking if one is having trouble speaking; it is much like asking a person who has cerebellar ataxia to remain calm while trying to walk a tightrope! Marital disharmony, in particular, comes into consideration with parents of stutterers; interestingly, there has been little systematic study of the incidence of divorce and/or separation among the parents of stutterers. Our clinical observations suggest that the divorce rate among the parents of stutterers is no greater than that of the average public; perhaps, the parents of stutterers are more likely to remain together and work out and/or tolerate their concerns within their marriage.

Psychologically, it is important to ascertain if clients seek services for themselves or for others. External prodding, as from a parent or spouse, may get a person in the therapy door, but it will not provide the effort level, initiative, and insight necessary to successfully complete therapy. Psychological concerns that hinder therapeutic progress consist of such things as being overly subjective about the problem (or unable to be objective about the problem even with our help), overly passive and/or consumer-oriented ("looking for the cure"), overly argumentative-intellectual about the problem ("deny emotions and explanation for behavior"), and so forth. Our experience has led us to become particularly concerned if during some preliminary exploring with the client or his or her parents, we broach a possible reason or explanation of behavior that needs changing and the client or parent does one or both of the following: (1) categorically or flatly denies that the reason or explanation has any validity or (2) provides a myriad of excuses for why the behavior occurred or is necessary or important. We have found that the denial and/or excuse means of coping with a problem is a very counterproductive mechanism and is, in our opinion, an indicator of less than positive prognosis. Later on in this book we discuss, in detail, psychological coping mechanisms (Vaillant 1977) and their possible implications for therapeutic management of stutterers and their associates. For now, however, let us leave it that psychological coping mechanisms are as important to the evaluation of stuttering as are the problems the stutterer and associates are coping with. Finally we come to that group of individuals (5 percent to 15 percent?) whose psychosocial concerns are of a degree and kind that warrant professional evaluation and counselling by trained psychiatrists or psychologists. These individuals, as Van Riper (1973) so aptly put it, seem to stutter ". . . at you with a gleam in their eye" and our only problem is being able to discern that gleam! The stuttering problem and all its manifold aspects seem, for a certain small percentage of stutterers, to fulfill unmet needs, and it is this group of clients who need to be referred to a professional counselor.

○ WHO IS AND WHO IS NOT REFERRED FOR THERAPY

After the completion of the evaluation comes the moment of truth: Should the client be seen for therapy and if so, what should be the form of such therapy? Obviously, there are no easy answers to such a question; however, there are some general guidelines that can be followed. Others have discussed some of the behaviors (for example, Ainsworth 1977; Adams 1977) we should watch for with the young child, and we think *two* such behaviors are of particular significance: (1) Is the child prolonging sounds (is this the most frequent disfluency type) and (2) Is the child avoiding or averting eye contact with listeners? When these two behaviors are apparent, the child is a good candidate for speech therapy. On the other hand, a child may exhibit some sound prolongations and avoidance of eye contact but predominately produce easy part-word repetitions and good eye contact with listeners; these children bear monitoring by means of follow-up evaluations. Finally, some children are doing nothing more than is normal for their chronological and developmental level, and the parents have to be so counselled. With these clients and parents, time spent in counselling and information sharing regarding normal childhood development and behavior is time well spent. Sometimes, with these parents, other concerns besides stuttering are the real concern, for example, inability to tell time and be punctual; inability to keep a tidy room; inability to read, write, and count; and so forth. More often than not, these parents are trying to speed up the pace of their child's development, or they are becoming overly concerned that a relative or neighbor's child can do this or that before or better than their child. The stuttering, therefore, becomes the focus whereas what really troubles them is that their child is "less than perfect." LeShan (1963), in a marvelous book discussing such normal parental concerns, says much that is of assistance to clinician and parent alike in understanding and dealing with these matters. The bottom line, so to speak, regarding referring or not referring children who stutter for speech therapy is that we want to avoid making a rush to judgment; that is, we need to exercise patience and care before we embark on an in-clinic therapy regimen for the child. On the other hand, children who have clearly developed a problem that maturation and parental counselling would not resolve need therapy. I have seen a child of four and a half years who definitely needs therapy while another of eight years may be appropriately dealt with through parental counselling and education. We need to consider not the age of the child with the problem but the age of the problem with the child.

With adults, the trilogy of therapy referrals goes like this: (1) those who clearly need therapy, (2) those who may need therapy, and (3) those whose problems do not warrant therapy for stuttering. Note that the third category assumes that the client may have a problem but that this problem is not stuttering. It may be speech apraxia, dialectical speech and language usage, psychoneurotic concerns, employment concerns, and so forth. We should not dismiss these other concerns out of hand but instead make the proper referrals to agencies more equipped and trained to deal with them.

The second category of referrals, those who may need therapy, are the fluent or relatively fluent stutterers, and their presence is an everyday reality in a college or hospital clinic. Although they may appear essentially fluent, they are very concerned about their speech and their ability to interact with others, particularly through verbal communication. These are the individuals, as mentioned before, that apparently have no problem but because they adamantly believe they have a problem, they have one! I have found that adult group therapy is beneficial for this type of client. It provides a forum to compare and contrast other problems as well as to learn more about speaking and to gain more reasonable standards for fluent verbal communication.

The first category, those who really need therapeutic assistance, are characterized by frequent within-word disfluencies (sound prolongations, sound-syllable repetitions and within-word pauses), frequent and persistent aversion of eye contact with listeners, avoidance of speaking situations, words, and sounds, strong personal identification as a stutterer, and labelling by close and casual acquaintances as a stutterer. These individuals can benefit from a combination of individual and group therapy with the more frequent sessions per week, the better. The group serves as a place to meet others with similar concerns, to learn from as well as share with them similar problems and questions, to feel that they are not "alone in the boat," to sort out everyday from specific concerns regarding stuttering, and to gain experience with verbal communication in a group situation. Obviously, individual therapy can be more closely tailored to the specific client as well as amplify topics brought up in group therapy.

Thus, we can see that for both the child and the adult who stutter, the decision to enter therapy is not a black and white decision. There is always the marginal situation where therapy may or may not be of assistance. Nothing precludes, however, trial therapy of three to six weeks in duration from being employed with the marginal clients to see if remediation has a chance of being beneficial. Remediation presupposes a thorough evaluation, and it is necessary to weigh all factors in coming to a conclusion for or against therapy. In this chapter we have tried to explore and share with you some of those factors which should be considered. In subsequent chapters we investigate considerations involved in the remediation of stuttering. Hopefully, the reader will see how our regimens for remediation flow or follow from our approaches to evaluation.

SUMMARY

Evaluating stuttering involves two general procedures: (1) interview of client and associates regarding attitudes, feelings, and beliefs concerning the problem and related matters and (2) subjective and objective assessment of speech fluency and related speech-language behavior, for example, speech articulation, language usage (receptive and expressive), voice quality, and so forth. Additional aspects such as reading, academic standings and progress, social maturity, gross/fine motor skills, cognitive abilities, and so forth should be evaluated according to the dictates of each individual case. Evaluation is a very important aspect of the remediation of stuttering because the nature of the problem will dictate the procedure used to remediate it.

Clinical evaluation of speech fluency necessitates that the clinician develop skills differentiating between-word (for example, phrase repetitions) from within-word (for example, sound repetitions) disfluencies as well as being able to determine the average frequency of each disfluency type per 10 or 100 words or syllables. The clinician will also need to become aware of the temporal components of speech: duration of each instance of stuttering, number of words spoken or read per minute, duration of within- and between-word pauses, length of time from the end of the client's statement to the beginning of parent's reply ("turn taking"), and so forth. Stuttering is a disruption in the forward flow of speech production; it is a disruption in the relatively rapid, smooth articulatory movements from one speaking posture to the next. Indeed, careful assessment of the temporal aspects of speech production is essential when evaluating stuttering. Any and all factors, whether external or internal to the client, that contribute to the client's temporal disruptions in their forward movement in speech production is something that the clinician must evaluate with regard to its potential contribution to the client's stuttering.

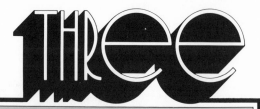

○ YOUNG CHILDREN WITH NO COMMUNI-
CATIVE CONCERNS, WHOSE PARENTS
ARE CONCERNED

○ CHILDREN WITH SOME STUTTERING
AND (UN)CONCERNED PARENTS

○ CHILDREN WHO CLEARLY STUTTER
AND PARENTS WHO ARE (UN)CON-
CERNED

○ REFERRALS TO OTHER PROFESSION-
ALS

○ GENERAL SUGGESTIONS REGARDING
PARENT COUNSELLING

○ SUMMARY

Remediation: young children who stutter

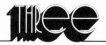

Some young children who stutter are eager and ready for speech therapy while others hang back and appear to resist the speech-language patholo-gist's every effort. Some of these youngsters appear to be quick studies who readily make and implement necessary change while others appear uncer-tain and confused about almost everything that goes on in therapy. Some young stutterers easily leave mom and dad and proceed into the therapy room while others kick and scream as if being led to the gallows! Truly, understanding the dynamics of which young stutterers are helpable, moti-vated, and able to benefit from speech and language remediation is as complicated as it is with older stutterers.

To complicate matters even further, the speech-language pathologist must also deal with parents in the remediation of the young stutterer. Parents, like their children, come in all sizes and shapes, and their idiosyn-cracies will influence therapeutic success. Parents are often unclear regard-ing their role in remediation of the young stutterers; some parents see little if any purpose being served by their involvement. We would like to empha-size, however, that all the good that is done in therapy can be offset, in a relatively short time, by parents who cannot or will not understand their role in their child's speech development. Parents, of course, are not the only problem; sometimes speech and language pathologists can be responsible for unduly engendering guilt or confusion in parents regarding their contri-butions to their child's speech and language problems. Parents of young children who stutter need support and encouragement to make and explore change. They do not need additional reprimands and chastisements for past and present, real and imagined transgressions against their children. As mentioned previously, LeShan (1963) discusses the role of parental guilt in the upbringing of children, and I believe that LeShan's thoughts are well worth reading by speech and language pathologists who need to consider parental guilt and what should and should not be done about it.

One other general consideration is whether speech and language therapy with the child should be *direct* or *indirect.* Van Riper (1973) and others have already covered this topic, but it is a topic that continually seems to plague speech and language pathologists who service young stutterers. Two issues, at least, are involved: (1) mentioning the label *stuttering* in the presence of the child and/or the parents of the child and (2) talking to the young child, in clear, but none the less direct terms, about talking (for example, Williams 1971). Both issues, we are cautioned by some, are better not broached since they are counterproductive to successful remediation. Up to a point we agree with this caution, but we need to recognize that young stutterers and their parents are not at the same level in their development of a problem. That is, we may label all such children as *incipient stutterers,* or *primary stutterers,* or *beginning stutterers,* or *young children beginning to stutter;* however, labelling all such children does not necessarily mean that all of these children are the same in terms of quantity and quality of problem. Perhaps, it is like saying that we have several fruits that on further examination break down into limes, lemons, grapefruit, and the like. All young children who stutter are not necessarily the same, even though they have certain commonalities. The indirect approach may be more feasible for some, whereas the "direct" procedure is more logical for others. At the risk of being redundant, it is not the age of the child with the problem, but the age of the problem with the child. There would appear to be little way an indirect approach (one that does not directly remediate speech fluency, in specific, and oral communication skills, in general) can have significant impact on a four year old's stuttering if that child is producing 30 percent disfluent speech with 90 plus percent of those disfluencies being sound prolongations! This does not mean, of course, that the *exact* direct procedures we would employ with an eighteen year old would be employed with this four year old; indeed, we would want to temper, modify, or drastically change certain of these procedures to make them suitable for the youngster. Nevertheless, we must recognize that the therapy we do is related to our evaluation of the stutterer. This evaluation, in turn, should be sensitive enough to discern the subcategories of apples, pears, plums, and peaches among the larger diagnostic category of fruit.

In the pages that follow, we examine three different, but related, kinds of young stutterers (see Andrews and Harris 1964 for further discussion of different subtypes of stutterers). We do not claim that this listing is exhaustive of all the young stutterers a speech-language pathologist might see, but our experience indicates that these groupings make up a large proportion of those young children labelled as stutterers. The groupings of children are based on our clinical experience with young stutterers evaluated and remediated in the Department of Communicative Disorders at Syracuse University. Table 3–1 offers some descriptive information regarding a group of these youngsters (N = 47) this author selected on the basis of their representativeness of youngsters he had clinically serviced for the problem of stuttering. For various reasons, not all children initially evaluated were subsequently seen for speech therapy at Syracuse University (for example, the family moved out of the area). However, enough of these children were remediated by this writer, his professional associates, or his graduate stu-

TABLE 3-1

Descriptive Information Regarding Youngsters Who Stutter
(N = 47) Initially Evaluated by the Present Author

These children were selected in terms of their representativeness of young stutterers whom the current author has evaluated and remediated. Severity of stuttering is based on the 7-point (0 = no stuttering to 7 = very severe stuttering) Iowa Scale for Rating Severity of Stuttering (Johnson and others, 1963).

Stutterings per 100 words spoken	
Mean	17.1
Range	0.0 to 40.0
Stuttering Severity Level	
Mean	3.5
Range	0.0 to 7.0
Disfluency Type	
Most Frequent	Part-word repetitions 27 of 47 clients
Least Frequent	Sound prolongations 16 of 32 clients (data not available for 15 clients)
Child's Age at Time of Initial Evaluation	
Mean	8.5 years
Range	3.3 to 12.8 years
Sex of Child	
Male	36
Female	11
Child's Position in Family	
First	15/47
Second	13/47
Third	7/47
Fourth	6/47
Fifth	5/47
Six	1/47
Parents Mean Age at Time of Initial Evaluation	
Mother	34.1 (range = 21 to 46)
Father	36.9 (range = 23 to 50)

dents under his supervision for certain observations to be made and impressions formulated.

The three categories of young stutterers are (1) children we evaluated as having no objective-subjective-communication problem, but whose parents or other adult listeners were concerned; (2) children we evaluated as having some objective-subjective-communication problem and whose parents and/or adult listeners may or may not have been concerned; and (3) children we evaluated as having a decided or clearly apparent problem and whose parents and/or adults may or may not have been, but probably were, concerned. The order in which we discuss these three categories is somewhat arbitrary; we begin with category (1) which predominately involves parental counselling and information sharing.

○ YOUNG CHILDREN WITH NO COMMUNICATIVE CONCERNS, WHOSE PARENTS ARE CONCERNED

Speech and language pathologists who work with young children should be aware of literature specifically addressed to remediation of young children who stutter (Luper and Mulder 1964; Williams 1971; Van Riper 1973). Likewise, the speech-language pathologist should be aware of and be prepared to share with parents available facts and figures publications (Johnson 1946; Ainsworth 1977; Cooper 1979). These latter publications can be given to parents to elaborate upon, reinforce, and clarify points made by the speech-language pathologist in counselling sessions. Such publications are not always read or understood by the parents, but with the clinician's encouragement and guidance, as well as further explanation and answering of questions, parents can gain valuable insights. Whatever the case, the speech and language pathologist should be thoroughly familiar with the contents of these self-help publications and be ready and willing to help parents grasp and implement their contents.

When a child is essentially fluent, that is, when the child's type and frequency of disfluency is within normal limits for the child's chronological and developmental age level, remediation of the child's speech fluency is contraindicated. This picture is made less clear, however, when the parents or other important adult listeners insist or strongly believe that a stuttering problem exists. In most cases, these parents are raising their first child, and they are generally, but not exclusively, younger parents (thirty years old and younger). They appear to want the best for their child and seem to expect, in a number of areas, that the child will achieve at high levels of performance, regardless of the child's ability. These parents fall into three different, but not necessarily mutually exclusive, camps:

1. Why can't Johnny be perfect (like I was)?
2. My husband (wife) is wrong and he (she) thinks I'm wrong about how to raise our child.
3. These problems run in the family.

The first camp, why can't Johnny be perfect, is the situation where the parent(s) seem to want their child to be perfect and they are frustrated because the child, like most humans, cannot achieve such perfection. These parents often tell you that they want their five-year-old son to be a doctor, a lawyer, or some other professional. Such parents seem to have trouble believing that their standards for their child are in error and therefore feel the problem must be produced or caused by the child. The child many times appears to be heavily monitored in terms of communication and social and academic development, and the parents seem quite demanding of and rigid in their standards for their child. These are the parents who need assistance in viewing their standards for child development and performance relative to other children of the same chronological and developmental age. They must be patiently, but firmly, instructed that their expectations for their child and for his or her speech and language development need to be evaluated and adjusted. As previously mentioned, booklets like those developed by Ainsworth (1977) and Cooper (1979) will assist in providing the parents with information and suggestions for change. We find that these parents can be helped if they will listen to reason; that is, they can be helped if they can entertain the notion that their standards for their child are less (or more) than desirable and that these standards need reevaluation and change. In some cases, referrals to psychologists and psychiatrists who specialize in child-family counselling may be the only way such change can be made. We have observed, however, that the child's problem is generally resolved when the parents' concern and standards for the child's performance can be reduced and brought into line with what is considered reasonable for a child the age of theirs.

Related to the why-can't-Johnny-be-perfect situation, is the situation where one parent thinks the other is wrong and vice versa. This is commonly seen where the wife *frequently* and *consistently* complains that the husband is too strict with the child. Neither parent seems to agree with the other in terms of the way in which the child should be raised (such disagreements are generally noticed when discipline is an issue) or how a child of their son's or daughter's age should speak, think, read, write, behave, play, and so forth. Such parents openly and frequently disagree about the raising of the child in front of the child. The key to this parental dilemma, like other parental dilemmas, is the *frequency* and *consistency* with which these problems exist. If the problems are so pervasive that arguments between parents are the rule, rather than the exception, the parents may need more than simple information sharing and informal counselling. Perhaps the child is the focal point for difficulties the mother and father have between themselves, and they take out their frustrations and anger with each other on the child. In some of these cases referral to appropriate psychological services may be appropriate. However, we have found that most of these parents will listen to reason and seriously try to minimize their differences when they come to realize that their difficulties may be adversely influencing the child. In such cases, where one parent may be convinced that the child is stuttering and the other may be diametrically opposed to this notion, the clinician should avoid giving the appearance of choosing sides. Persistence on the part of the clinician in helping the parents to see their child as he or she really is, is important. Continued reiteration of basic child development information is also of import. The speech-language pathologist must persevere in these matters if he or she expects to move these parents in the right direction. The clinician should try to (1) be persistent, (2) convey respect for the parents, and (3) express the fact that the parents love their child. If the clinician can do all three, it is amazing the change these parents can and do make and the degree to which the child's communication "problem" can be resolved. The parents, like all of us, want to do the right thing and with support and a little guidance from thoughtful professionals, can do more and more of the right things for their child and themselves.

Another situation occurs when one or both parents say that the child's stuttering stems from the fact that stuttering runs in one or both of their families. These parents give the appearance of waiting for the other shoe to drop; they have been looking since the child began to speak for signs of stuttering, and they have finally found them. Many times one or both parents will mention the horrible stuttering problem of an Uncle Ralph or Sister Kate and how they hope that their Johnny does not end up the same way. These parents seem to have high expectations for their child's speech, language, and fluency development even in the face of evidence that their child may be developing at his or her own normal, albeit slow, pace. The parents have many old persons' tales about what causes stuttering and what makes it better or worse. They may bring up the issue of whether stuttering is a result of a physical flaw or a psychological problem. These parents probably need information regarding normal child development in general and communication development in specific. They may begin to shop around from one clinician to another until they find one who will agree that their child has a fluency problem. It is important, particularly with this type of parent, to quickly establish your credibility and concern for their child. Your patience will be tested because you will have to continually reiterate what you believe the parents need to consider to make appropriate change. Although recent work (Kidd and others 1977) suggests some degree of genetic involvement with stuttering, this does not mean that the parents and clinician must throw up their hands and give in. Indeed, knowing that their child may be predisposed to reacting to psychosocial or communicative stress by repeating or prolonging speech segments (that is, stuttering) should make these parents work all the harder to minimize those elements in their interactions with the child which may be contributing to their child's tendency to stutter.

When all is said and done, counselling parents about their child's apparently nonexistent stuttering problem is both remediative and preventative. You try, through information sharing, discussion, and counselling, to help the parents provide for their child a home environment conducive to optimal development of speech fluency and related behavior, such as emotions, feelings, attitudes, and so forth. During this time, the parents may want you to "therapize" the child—the degree to which they insist on this therapy may be an indirect measure of the degree to which they are abdicating their role in the problem. Perhaps, seeing the child for informal play therapy (see, Axline 1947; Murphy and Fitzsimmons 1960; Van Riper 1973) or for general speech and language stimulation may assuage the parents while you discuss with them what they may do to change their interactions with and expectations of their child. Many times, directly after the initial evaluation, when the parents have just been interviewed and the problem is fresh in their minds, is a good time for a thirty to sixty minute information sharing session. Sometimes this initial postevaluation findings and recommendations session is all these parents need to significantly diminish their concerns. Make sure, before these parents leave the first time, that they have your clinical phone number and address and that they truly feel that they can call you (we specifically tell them, "Feel free to call") if they have further questions or concerns. It is important to keep the door to your clinic open. Do not "lock" the parents out; let them know you want to maintain contact and welcome their calls. Try to provide parents with a sense that someone is available to help and that the parents themselves have the ability to positively change. In these situations, we attempt to set up a reevaluation four to twelve months later. Such reevaluations also allow us to monitor the child's speech and the parents' actual ability to positively change. Maintain the contact with these parents, not as a means to extend your professional preciousness, but as a way for these parents to contact you at times when they are concerned. Keeping in touch with the parents reduces their feeling of helplessness and "being alone in the boat"; your suggestions and insights may well be the only voice of reason the parents hear, and they need that. Besides, you are not emotionally involved with the child and can be objective in your suggestions. We also feel it is important for clinicians to know and understand what parenting books the parents have and/or are reading. The young parent raising a first child usually reads such books as those by Spock (1946), those published by Gesell and associates (for example, Ilg and Ames 1960), or the more recent ones like that of Dodson (1970). The speech-language pathologist should read and be familiar with these books and develop an understanding of the types of written inputs many parents turn to when they have questions and concerns about the general well-being of their child.

○ CHILDREN WITH SOME STUTTERING AND (UN)CONCERNED PARENTS

Children who are beginning to evidence within-word disfluencies more frequently than adult listeners believe they should are a difficult lot to evaluate and remediate. These children generally, but not always, exhibit no apparent awareness of speech disfluency problem. Their disfluencies are marked by cyclical changes; one day (or week, or month) they are "good" (that is, they do not stutter) and the next, "bad" (that is, they stutter quite frequently). Most of their disfluencies are *easy* in that they exhibit little signs of physical tension associated with these disfluencies. Most of the disfluencies seem to be either part-word or monosyllabic whole-word repetitions with less frequent sound prolongations. The clinician may notice that these children have subtle or not so subtle problems with articulation, language, or psychosocial development. Based on our experience, tests like the Vineland Test of Social Maturity suggest social maturation within normal limits, and other tests like the Peabody Picture Vocabulary Test or the Ammon's Quick Test indicate that vocabulary recognition is within normal limits (the Quick Test results are highly correlated to a full-scale WISC). We have clinically observed that some of these children may have slightly slower or less precise fine motor coordination of fingers and speech musculature than normal; however, in most regards these children seem within normal limits.

Parents may have brought their child to you because others said the child has a problem or because they themselves believe the child has a problem. In either case, parent involvement in therapy will be necessary to help to develop an environment which optimizes opportunities for the child to develop normal speech fluency. Parents must not be made to feel unduly guilty about their role in the problem, but they should understand their role and the things they can do to help and change.

If the child's speech fluency problem is secondary to another problem (for example, language delay), the other problem may need more immediate attention. We have noticed in the clinic that some children whose language seemed delayed and/or deviant became more disfluent when their language actually began to improve (with or without speech-language therapy)! This association between positive change in language and increases in speech disfluency seems particularly noticeable when the child is around five or six years of age. It is not uncommon to see a child with some stuttering to have a mean length of utterance (MLU) (Brown 1973) roughly appropriate for his or her chronological age, but whose mastery of particular grammatical morphemes (that is, morphemes whose main purpose is to modify meaning of content words or to more specifically indicate relation of content words) is less than appropriate for this stage of language development. For example, the use of *be* as a copula verb (the *is* of "She is fired" and the *are* of "You are president") may be omitted by some children who stutter who are at Brown's stage IV of language development. We are not saying that all of these children who stutter have language problems, or that they all exhibit lack of appropriate grammatical morphemes, or that language problems cause stuttering. However, delays in language development (Johnston and Schery 1976) do occur with some children who stutter, and as such, these problems need to be assessed. In fact, if we believe a child's speech disfluencies are secondary to delays and deviance in language development, it is my recommendation that language skills need attention prior to remediation of fluency. I say this particularly when the speech disfluencies are of an easy, part- and whole-word repetition variety; however, frequent sound prolongations associated with visible and audible signs of physical and psychological tension, even when associated with language concerns, are suggestive of more direct therapeutic intervention with fluency.

Articulatory difficulties often go along with language problems which may accompany the disfluency problem. We find articulatory difficulties to be especially hard to deal with when they accompany speech disfluency; of course, there are articulatory problems, and then there are articulatory problems. A slight distortion of an /s/, or perhaps an /l/, is no real problem and can be ignored as the clinician proceeds to deal with the disfluency; however, multiple articulation errors with omissions, and substitutions, as well as distortions, are problematic. We are very reluctant to remediate a child's articulation errors when that child is beginning to evidence more frequent than usual within-word disfluencies. Perhaps this is overly conservative on my part, but I have a rationale based on experience, observation, and philosophy. My rationale is that these children do not need further instruction in which sounds are problems or difficult to produce. That is, they do not need further instruction in how to work at, force out, or be careful with their problem sounds. They do not need to learn concern, fear, fright, avoidance, and struggle when confronted with the production of certain sounds. Indeed, they already seem to have these ideas or are at least on the road to developing such notions! What these children need is assistance in developing more easy, less physically forced means of initiating speech and not careful, cautious and overly articulated productions of sounds. These children already seem to have developed a strategy towards speech production which we interpret as ". . . speech is hard, speech takes work, and thus I'll use force (or avoid) to speak" (Bloodstein 1975). Unfortunately, too many of our good intentions to assist some of these children with their articulation difficulties backfire on us when the youngsters just learn more sounds to fear and more and better ways to physically tense up and push out speech segments (see Dell 1980 for further discussion of ways to deal with these issues with the school-age stutterer).

With the child who is stuttering somewhat, the clinician has two basic choices: (1) bring the child in for therapy or (2) observe the child through the periodic reevaluation route. Neither way, I believe, is completely satisfactory. With the first approach, you run the risk of boring the child and the parents with therapy since you may not get improvement fast enough or in sufficient quantity to maintain motivation and satisfaction with therapy. With the second approach, you run the risk of having the child's fluency problem or environment deteriorate. We bring the child and his or her parents in if the parents understand it is initially for a trial period of, say, three to six weeks. If the child and parents seem to benefit from this trial therapy, fine; if not, we cancel and put the client and family into a hold pattern in which we observe through periodic reevaluations, phone calls to parents and school, and school and home visits (if possible). It is too easy to make a rush to judgment and bring the child in for therapy when parents and others are pushing for remediation. This is where your professional judgment must enter: Is the child emotionally, communicatively, and otherwise ready for therapy?

If we do bring children in for therapy, the first session, at least, is spent in getting to know the child, setting down rules of the road for the therapy sessions, and continually assessing whether the child's infrequently produced speech disfluencies warrant therapy. Rather than work on specific sounds, or words, or situations, we try to help the child, if this is indicated, develop an appropriate strategy to initiate speech. Some of the children also need to learn how to listen and wait their turn in a conversation. They may also need to learn that when they do have a turn to speak, this is not always an opportunity for a ten to fifteen minute monologue. They may need practice in logically and sequentially describing events and telling stories. Van Riper (1973) and others have described the types of play activities one may use with these children; I have found it instructive for parents to see us play with and talk with their child. Although parents will frequently say, "I simply don't have the time to spend playing with Bobby that you do," or "We don't have at home all those nice toys," or "I don't like to play with children," we try to emphasize to the parent the *quality,* rather than the *quantity,* of our play interactions with the child. We point out such things as a clinician's unconditional, positive regard for the child, the clinician's listening to the content of the child's utterances, the clinician's clear, but firm, setting down of rules, and the clinician's instructions on how to do a task (frequently, we find, parents think that telling Johnny to make his bed is sufficient when they have never really spent time instructing and showing Johnny how to make his bed).

For a child whose part-word disfluencies are inconsistent, but whose situation strongly suggests continued negative development, we may and do become fairly direct. Using Williams' (1971) concept of *hard* and *easy* speech, we instruct the child to identify hard speech in our speech and his or her speech and then to learn strategies to insure more easy speech. One caution, however, is parents who take the terms *hard* and *easy* and rewrite them into their own vocabulary and usage, using these terms in phrases like, "Stop that hard speech!" We never cease to be amazed at how some parents can continually and consistently selectively attend to only the negative aspects of their child's behavior. It is not uncommon for these parents to ask me whether they can say to their child in nice, positive tones, "That's it, that's good easy speech!" Yet, these same parents never ask me whether they can say, "Stop that hard speech this instant!" We explain to the parents that a little praise now and then, anything to build their child's positive self-image, must be correct and should be good for them and the child. Parents are generally anxious to help their child, and such help seems to be viewed by parents as an active, direct involvement. They want to *do* something to help their child. Such parents seem to find it difficult to accept the fact that not doing something is actually doing something! The terms *hard* and *easy* speech are nice, simple terms with minimal negative connotations associated with them (Williams 1971). These terms may be used by the clinician to help children (if this seems appropriate) identify instances of hard and easy speech in their and others' speech; these terms can also be used to describe speech targets that children can aim towards. We do not want the parent to simply substitute *hard* for *stuttering* and then go around reprimanding, correcting, nagging, or badgering the child regarding his hard speech. This defeats the purpose of the term and its use with the child; here the child's parent is doing something to help the child which is clearly not helping. That is, the parent's advice to the child becomes part of, rather than solution for, the problem. Parents must be assisted to see that such active helping may have to wait until both they and their child are at a more advanced state of therapy progress.

Establishing fluency with a young child who is somewhat more disfluent than normal can be a problem but not an insurmountable one. As has been discussed by Van Riper (1973) and others, engaging the child in low-level types of verbal conversation can often times help. We are particularly receptive to Stocker's (1976) notion of level of demand in which she has developed five categories of questions that require different levels of linguistic and cognitive formulation (see Conture and Caruso 1978). Surely, future work will refine these levels of demand and probably expand on their number and quality; however, for the present, the idea of relatively systematically controlling the child's utterance by the nature of the question one asks has intuitive appeal. One would surely not restrict an entire therapy session to questions of only one type, for example, "Is the ball big or little? blue or red? hard or soft? on the table or off the table?" Such questions could be used to elicit speech from the child once the child is talking, and the types of questions we ask can control, influence, and shape the child's fluency as well as reinstitute fluency after a period when the child has become disfluent. One might even be able to find types of questions that routinely, for a particular child, elicit fluency or disfluency and instruct parents in the use or avoidance of such questions, as the case may be. Obviously, our knowledge of the cognitive and linguistic development of young children who stutter, and those who do not, is still less than complete. Much more basic and applied research is needed in this area.

In some instances, a child who is frequently disfluent may be routinely picked on by other children and siblings. We have witnessed this ourselves inside as well as outside the clinic. This ridicule and mocking must be mitigated. If the children who pick on the disfluent youngster are the child's siblings, then the parents must intervene. Out of sight and sound of the child who is disfluent, the parents must take the sibling(s) aside and try, as patiently, clearly, and nonjudgmentally as possible, to explain that such teasing is neither polite nor kind to their brother or sister. The parents can help the sibling see that everybody has strengths and weaknesses and that their brother or sister makes mistakes sometimes when he or she talks. These mistakes are no reason to tease and make fun of the child. We all make mistakes in something we do; for example, we do not always throw or catch a ball right; we do not always spell every word right or print or write each letter correctly; we sometimes trip going up and down the stairs or fall off our bicycle; and so forth. The parent can help the sibling understand that mistakes are the normal part of growing up (indeed, of living) and that their brother or sister simply makes mistakes when he or she talks, but that with time and encouragement these mistakes will become fewer and fewer. This polite but firm parental lecture may have to be delivered several times, always out of sight and sound of the child who is disfluent, and in extreme cases, the clinician may have to talk with the siblings. We have had several cases where we have had to talk to other siblings about teasing, correcting, reprimanding, and harassing. Sometimes these older siblings were only ten or twelve years of age or slightly younger, but in at least three instances, these older children were between sixteen and twenty years of age! We have also noticed that neighborhood children pick up clues on how to react to the young child who stutters by how the parents and siblings react. If the siblings have an accepting and noncritical attitude towards the child who stutters, chances are (remember, we said chances and not certainty) the neighborhood kids will react likewise. If the child is in preschool, nursery, or early elementary school and teasing becomes an issue, the teacher may have to intervene. Van Riper (1973) and Williams (1971) discuss the names and difficulties encountered by the disfluent child who may be teased in school. Van Riper (1973, pp. 434–435) provides excellent suggestions for dealing with such schoolyard and classroom teasing. Unfortunately, as anyone who has *continually* experienced verbal teasing can attest, "names can really hurt you." Parental concerns over such teasing are often times very real and pervasive, and such concerns need to be discussed and positive steps taken to alleviate them.

One thing that we note with some of these children is their basic difficulty with verbal expression. Now before you start saying, "Where are the data?" let me reiterate that I said *some* and not all. Furthermore, for lack of a better term, I referred to *verbal expression* to describe such things as the amount of time spent talking, the precise moment when to begin talking, logically organizing thoughts into language, knowing when is a good time to interrupt people who are talking, and knowing how to appropriately get listener attention. These subtleties of verbal expression (see, for example, Bates 1976; Rees 1980; for an overview of the pragmatics of language usage) are seemingly unclear to some of the young children who are beginning to be disfluent. They may monologue at the dinner table (to everybody's discomfort and utter boredom); they may seem to "put the cart before the horse" in many of their expressions; they may, instead of waiting their turn, repeat sounds, syllables, words, and phrases to gain listener attention, hold the floor of a conversation, or interrupt an already ongoing conversation, and yet seem to expect no one to interrupt them after they have begun talking.

We say these things based on clinical observations of the children, parental reports of their child's verbal interaction traits, and in-home observations of these same children. Now, it must be confessed that many other children who do not stutter also do these same things, but we are not sure of the frequency and consistency of this behavior on the part of the nonstutterers. Further, we are sure some parents have a shorter fuse for such undesirable verbal expression traits than the average parent. Likewise, siblings who are also trying to gain the speaking floor and their parents' attention may not be too tolerant of a brother or sister who takes up more than his or her fair share of the time or who takes what they think is too long a time to begin speaking or to get to the point of their speaking. These verbal annoyances must be dealt with in therapy and explored with the parents to see if they exist and if they do, how the family is reacting. The child's inability in these areas leads, in my mind, to one of the many Catch-22s of stuttering. For example, the child who takes too long to get to the point of his or her topic and who tends to monologue once he or she does get the speaking floor becomes the child that other children, and parents, and adults find less and less enjoyable to verbally interact with. However, if this child gets less and less opportunity to practice verbal expression, his or her skills in this area have little chance for being exercised, and thus the child remains less than adequately developed in these areas. This means that he or she still gets called on less frequently to speak! Such vicious cycles, with which the problem of stuttering abounds, must be identified at an early age and changed before they develop into consistent, undermining problems which contribute to the maintenance and perpetuation of stuttering.

One last suggestion that I give to parents of these children is to talk more and read more with their children. Van Riper's (1973) cautions in this area are well taken; however, it is my experience that with patience and persistence on the part of the speech-language pathologist, parents can learn, and even come to enjoy, reading to their children. Reading to a child can become a family ritual-tradition that closes out the day in a relaxed, mutually satisfying way. The parent gets a chance to talk to the child, and the child has an opportunity to listen to and ask questions of the parents. Problems in this area, however, do exist, as Van Riper noted, and the speech-language pathologist must be familiar with them if this home suggestion is to work. First, the parent should pick out books and stories that the child can understand, relate to, and enjoy. One mother of a five year old could not understand why her son seemed bored with her reading of a *National Geographic* article on the Apollo space mission! Help the parent learn what kinds of stories, and print, and pictures a child of their child's age might understand and enjoy. Dodson (1970) presents a very comprehensive listing of books and stories appropriate for various ages of children. Secondly, do not give the parents the impression that they must buy these books themselves; encourage them to visit local libraries and to bring their child with them. Be patient and supportive, and tell them that with time and experience, their child will select books independently, but that in the beginning the parent will have to do much of the selecting. Third, pick the parent, whether mother or father, that you think has the most patience and interest in reading *aloud* to the child. The athletic father or the extremely quiet mother may not be your best bet; try to figure out who would be the best (but not perfectionistic) out loud reader and who would have the most patience for same. Fourth, encourage the parent to read in a calm, relatively unhurried fashion and to expect, even encourage, the child to interrupt and ask questions. Indeed, if the parent simply cannot tolerate the child's interruptions for questions and comments, that parent is a poor risk for a reader. We have been able, however, employing patience and persistence, to help parents like this to learn and modify their abilities in this area so that they can become good, or at least, adequate oral readers. Encourage parents to read every day to their children, but let them know it is all right to skip an evening or day when they are just not in the mood. We have found reading to children to be an excellent vehicle for parent-child sharing; for providing a good adult model of easy, relaxed speaking; and for giving practice to the child in hearing an adult voice speaking to them for a period of time (the very thing they experience in school classrooms every day). We think that it is clear that such reading is also a stimulant for the child's vocabulary development and that it also helps the child to learn to read for enjoyment and entertainment. If we can believe what we read about television's being a less than positive influence on our children (Winn 1977), then the more reading we expose our children to and that they do themselves, the better.

Most of the preceding is directed at parents and parent interaction with children because I believe that children who have some objective problems with speech disfluencies, accompanied by possible parental concern over such problems, can still most effectively be dealt with through the parents. At the risk of being redundant, let me say that this assumes that the child is mostly producing, in a relatively nontense fashion, part-word repetitions, that the child's eye contact with listeners, when the child speaks, is within normal limits, and that the child appears to be basically unaware of a speech problem. As Ainsworth (1977) points out, as sound prolongations, in particular, start to appear more frequently and eye contact starts to fall off (probably less than 50 percent of the time the child's eyes are in contact with his or her listener's), we must begin to work more and more with the child. As always, however, there are the children who fall in the cracks, children who are exhibiting some sound prolongations but whose eye contact is not seriously diminished. It is these children who present us with many of our most perplexing clinical situations because they are in-between and we are not sure which way they are going to progress. It would be nice if we could find signs like, for example, middle-ear concerns, which would suggest that these children, for reasons that are still unclear, are progressing in a negative direction. Hopefully, more basic and applied research can be undertaken and funded to discover which variables predict positive and negative change in speech disfluencies. Why implement therapy regimens when with time and positive parental intervention some of the children we see, who are beginning to stutter, will improve on their own? Unfortunately, we are still missing the data that would allow us to make such decisions based on a more solid foundation.

○ CHILDREN WHO CLEARLY STUTTER AND PARENTS WHO ARE (UN)CONCERNED

These children are frequently producing within-word disfluencies (probably in excess of six within-word disfluencies per 100 words spoken), and adults (most likely, but not necessarily, the parents) notice and report these disruptions. Interestingly, parents are most concerned about (1) the part-word repetitions and (2) concomitant nonspeech behavior, for example, facial grimaces. Facial grimaces, in particular, will many times be the final straw that makes parents call and set up an evaluation for their child. Likewise, some parents seem to breathe a sigh of relief when their child begins to prolong more than repeat, even though our clinical intuition and experience suggest that the child's stuttering problem is worsening. Unfortunately, some professionals, with not enough experience or interest in stuttering, will use up precious time in the beginning of the child's development of stuttering and only refer to a more qualified professional when the child is showing signs of a worsening problem. However, our observation of this problem is not meant to nor will it cure these or other worldly woes. It merely serves as a comment on their occurrence and a hope for a better tomorrow.

A child who is frequently stuttering to the point where direct therapeutic intervention is necessary is a child who needs a supporting and encouraging therapy environment. We cannot emphasize this point enough: We, as speech-language pathologists, should not pester the child the same way the parents and other children may be pestering him or her. Too often we tend to talk to children in an "old wine in new bottles" vocabulary that does nothing more than change the name while the game remains the same: *Stop that stuttering!* Many of these children do not want to hear, see, and feel what their stuttering is like; indeed, they want to avoid all mention of and confrontation with it as if they are ostriches with their heads in the sand. Getting them to do these things will take patience, time, and encouragement. Ideally, they would like some procedure, or technique, or passive cure, or device that would take their stuttering away from them. It is appropriate from the beginning to help the children see that there are different ways we can begin to speak and that some ways sound and feel better than others. I like to use analogies with my clients so that I can take the complex task of speaking and break it down into terms and objects that make sense to the client. Since speech production is so complex, it takes years to gain familiarity with its many aspects, and we should, therefore, not be surprised that the lay client has difficulty grasping what he or she is *doing* to interfere with speech.

One analogy I like to use with youngsters is what I call the garden hose analogy (see Figures 3–1 and 3–2). Most children have played with and used a garden hose with a nozzle, and thus the analogy generally works. I explain the three parts of interest: the faucet on the side of the house, the garden hose itself attached to the faucet, and the nozzle on the end of the hose. We first talk about the garden hose and its parts and how the parts work separately and together as a unit. We next talk about how we can make the water flow through the hose and how we can shut off its flow or slow it down. For example, we could turn the water off or slow its flow by turning the faucet at the house, or we could bend the hose, or we could turn the nozzle. After the child seems to understand how the garden hose works (a real nozzle attached to a short length of real hose makes this more alive, but some

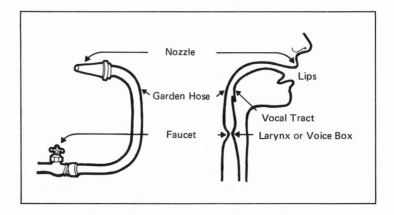

FIGURE 3–1 A lateral view of the supraglottal and glottal structures with their analogous parts of a garden hose-nozzle-faucet is presented The lips are equated with the nozzle of the hose in that both can be constricted to stop or modify airflow (lips) or water stream (nozzle). The vocal tract is analogized with the flexible, bendable garden hose in that both can be manipulated in such a way (the garden hose can be kinked or bent, and the vocal tract can have the tongue partially or completely occlude airway) as to impede or modify the airflow or water stream. Finally, the larynx or vocal folds (housed in voice box) are equated with the faucet in that both can be constricted or adjusted to stop or modify airflow or water stream. This analogy helps the young child identify the nature and function of each part of the vocal mechanism and the means by which his or her strategies to interfere with speech take place.

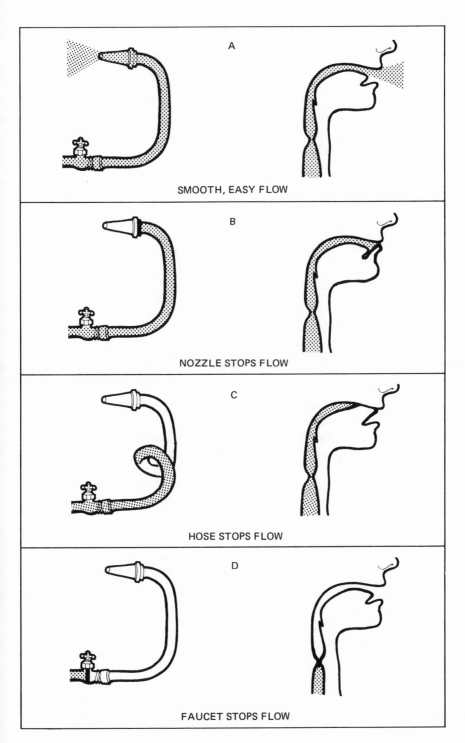

A

SMOOTH, EASY FLOW

B

NOZZLE STOPS FLOW

C

HOSE STOPS FLOW

D

FAUCET STOPS FLOW

FIGURE 3-2 (see page 58 for legend)

youngsters become too attentive to the hose—this calls for clinical judgment), we begin to discuss the similarities between the garden hose situation and our speech behavior. We talk about the larynx (voice box) as the faucet, and our throat and tongue as the garden hose, and our lips as the nozzle. We then practice "closing off the water" with our voice box, tongue, and lips. Having children take a deep breath and then hold it with their mouths open gives them an idea how the faucet or voice box stops the flow. Conversely, having children take a deep breath and hold it with lips closed and cheeks puffed out gives them the idea of how the nozzle or lips stop the flow. Having them hold the /s/ and then gradually stop air flowing through the constriction by raising the tongue and touching the palate gives them the idea how the hose or tongue stops the flow. We play with these various postures and *water stoppers,* or *flow stoppers,* or *air stoppers* until we feel the child has the idea or has had all the fun that he or she can stand!

We next introduce the idea of *air stoppers* in the child's actual speech by having the child observe us slow or stop the airflow through use of the nozzle, hose, or faucet. We then encourage the child to do the same on selected words and sounds. For example, the word-initial /b/ in the word *ball* could be used to demonstrate air stoppage at the level of the nozzle; the world-initial /k/ in the word *key,* for the level of the hose; and a word-initial vowel like /i/ in the word *eat,* for the level of the faucet. Laryngeal constriction or its converse, abduction, is a most difficult concept to get across to children (or adults, for that matter). As mentioned before, you can reinforce or explain the idea of air stopping at the larynx by having children hold their breath with the mouth open. The fact that the laryngeal area is not particularly rich in sensation, that its activity is invisible to the naked eye, and that children have no real good picture of what the larynx looks like or consists of makes this task all the more difficult. Unfortunately, for some children whose stuttering is a real problem and concern, laryngeal involve-

---

FIGURE 3–2 The four aspects of this figure (A, B, C, and D) depict the nature and function of vocal tract during fluent and stuttered speech. The smooth easy flow of air (A) for fluent speech strategies also shows how water flows through a garden hose in such a procedure. Naturally, during normal speech, the state of affairs depicted in A would be continually changing, but the idea of smooth, sequential movement from one speech posture to the next to produce a continuous flow of speech would still be apparent. In the first interfering situation (B), the client contacts too long and with too much pressure on the lips and dams the airflow in much the same way as the nozzle on the hose when tightened would stop water flowing from the hose. In the next inappropriate strategy (C), the person is seen contacting the hard palate with too much tension for too long which dams airflow in an analogous way to a kink in a garden hose blocking water from flowing. Finally, the vocal folds can be constricted (D) in such a way to impede airflow, much like turning a faucet off will impede water from flowing from the vocal tract. What is not easy to analogize is the inappropriate laryngeal strategy of opening the vocal folds (see Conture, McCall, and Brewer 1977). It is also possible for the three inappropriate strategies (B, C, D) to be combined in a variety of ways to interfere with speaking. In fact, such combinations of strategies are probably closer to the reality of the situation than the present examples which were independently presented for the purposes of clear explication.

ment is a major aspect of the peripheral manifestation of their stuttering. Indeed, some of these children, in the interim between the listener's question and the child's response, seem to take a deep breath and hold it with the larynx as if to prepare themselves for the task of speaking. This response must be mitigated if the child is to have a chance for significant improvement.

Laryngeal, vocal tract, or lip closure during speech leads to some degree of aerodynamic back pressure (Netsell 1973) and normal feelings of muscle tension-tonus. Obviously, when these closures are too long or too tight, associated back pressures and muscle tensions will not feel appropriate. It is my guesstimation that the "feelings of pressure . . . tightness in the chest" that children and adults who stutter report are these unusually high levels of air back pressures. I am separating out these aerodynamic events from those autonomic events associated with sympathetic nervous system discharge, for example, heart palpitation, lightness or heaviness feeling in the stomach, flushed feelings, and sweating palms (see, Guyton 1971; Turner 1969; Brutten and Shoemaker 1967). I try to help the child understand (to take some of the mystery out of the problem) that these feelings of pressure come from something he or she is doing. We revert back to the garden hose analogy and say that a quick closure of the nozzle makes the garden hose stiffen and maybe even jump in our hand. This stiffening or movement results from water pressure or the fact that the water is suddenly dammed up and has nowhere to go so it pushes out the sides of the flexible garden hose. This water behaves in much the same way as the air which the child suddenly dams up, with the compressed volume of air exerting pressure within the respiratory and vocal tract and causing feelings of tightness. We try to make the child see that there are reasons why he or she feels tight and constricted and that these feelings can be changed by doing different things.

If the child appears to get the general gist of what he or she does that interferes with speaking, seems to be able to describe and identify this interfering behavior, and appears willing to make the necessary changes, we move on to the next stage. Here too, I use analogies to get the child and parents to see what the child must do to increase speech fluency. Two analogies I use operate on the same theme: Speech involves a movement from one sound to the next. The first analogy involves pretending a frog or the child is jumping from one lily pad to the next to cross a stream. We pretend that each pad is a letter of a short word like *baby* and that we must hop from the bank to the first pad, then to the next pad, and so on until we reach the other bank. If we stay too long on a pad, if we jump on the pad hard with both feet (that is, if we prolong the sound), we will get wet, or go to the bottom of the creek, or have trouble smoothly and easily getting across the stream, or saying the word. Likewise, if we hop up and down on the pad (that is, repeat the sound) and do not move on to the next pad, we will also get wet, or go to the bottom of the creek, or have trouble smoothly and easily getting across the stream, or saying the word. In either case, we cannot easily, and smoothly, and quickly get across the stream if we land on one pad and stay there or jump up and down. Essentially the same idea is conveyed by another analogy where a floating barrel bridge, each barrel tied to the other with rope, is used to cross a stream. Here, too, a barrel that is jumped on hard and stood on or repeatedly jumped up and down on will keep us from getting across the stream or from producing the word.

For older children or adults, who would naturally scorn the perceived juvenile nature of the lily pad or barrel bridge analogies, we use our four fingers and thumb in much the same way. Here each finger is a letter or sound of a short word and my thumb, the tongue, or speech system produces each letter or sound. When the thumb is moved smoothly, sequentially, and easily from one finger to the next, I tell the client and relatives that this is like fluent speech. Stuttering, I explain, is much like my pressing for too long with too much force between my thumb and one finger (a prolongation) or repeatedly contacting the thumb and one particular finger (a part-word repetition). These analogies, of course, will not cure anyone in and of themselves, but they serve as a common ground of understanding and provide essential insights for the young client into what he or she does that interferes with speech and what it is necessary to change.

One of the fundamental problems with assisting children to do more and more things that normally fluent speakers do when they speak (Williams 1971) is that the child cannot really see what it is that he or she is doing that is facilitative or inhibitory to fluent speech. That is, when the child is learning to hold the crayon or pencil for writing, the child can readily visualize most of the correct hand postures and positions and to some extent the necessary movements and coordinations for writing. Likewise, most sports the child is learning can be readily visualized, practiced, and compared to a model. Speech, on the other hand, is for most intents and purposes invisible to the naked eye; that is, you really cannot watch the necessary movements for speech as you can, say those of tennis. In a sense, our young clients are as baffled by the how and why of speech production and movements as we may be by our heart movements. Surely we know the heart pumps blood and that it beats, but could we really describe the physical movements and contractions and configurations of our heart at work? We would have the same trouble as our clients because our speech and our heart are essentially out of sight, out of mind. For most of us, speech and cardiac behavior are automatic events that we give little thought to: We simply speak, and our heart simply beats. For children who stutter, however, some knowledge of how they speak and how they interfere with speaking is crucial in order for them to improve their speech fluency.

Acoustic and videotape recordings are means to the end of showing the child how he or she is speaking. Mirrors and clinician imitation are other forms. However, all such work must be done with caution and with a sensitivity towards the particular child's needs. Some children are excellent at discussing and demonstrating speech behavior and disfluency in the abstract but become very emotional and resist or refuse to cooperate when actual speech behavior is touched, or visualized, or heard. These children need time and patience on the part of the clinician because they are not going to get over these feelings of fear, avoidance, and denial in a hurry. Sometimes actually showing these children a model of the vocal tract or the larynx and allowing them to explore and ask questions about the model is helpful. They may be encouraged to ask questions about their own speech structures. Anything to mitigate the mystery surrounding their speech behavior and the structures that produce it is desirable. Of course, any approach with children must be done with an eye towards the child's level of understanding, experience, and ability to remember and assess complex concepts. And while there is a danger of being too intellectual with a young stutterer, clinicians, particularly younger clinicians with minimal experience with youngsters, must also guard against the opposite: oversimplification. An eight-year-old child in the third grade is not exactly receptive to approaches that would be used with a preschool stutterer. It is an important rule to remember to take children at the level they present rather than the level you think they should present or that they usually present.

Modifying the speech disfluency of a child who stutters is a balancing act. One must balance the necessity for speech change against the desire not to develop more and greater speech concerns and fears. Being calm and collected with the parents and child, no matter what their level of excitement or emotionality, is a first step. A second step is to help the child explore, in a general way, speech behavior and different ways in which people talk. Next, children are given a few descriptive phrases and words to help them begin to understand speech and their own speaking behaviors. Phrases like *hard and easy speech, stopping the air from flowing or coming out, easy movement from one sound to the next,* and the like serve as guides or aides to children in their perception of their own speech. All the while, the parents are conferred with so that they understand the short-and long-term goals in therapy and any intermediate steps. If the clinician expects little visible change during a particular phase of therapy, the clinician should tell the parent so. Likewise, if a subtle but positive change is occurring that the parent may not notice, the clinician should point out such a change to the parent. Involving the parents in therapy (a topic that warrants more space than these pages allow) cannot be underestimated. Parents have a need and a right to know what is going on, when they should be justifiably concerned, and when their concerns are less appropriate.

The moment of stuttering or the instance of stuttering is still an unclearly described event from a physiological point of view; however, important strides are being made to describe and quantify such physiology (Adams 1974; Conture, McCall, and Brewer 1977; Freeman and Ushijima 1978). At the risk of jumping the gun on this description, we state our hunch regarding the key behavior that must be changed before the moment of stuttering is changed. We make this prediction based on our yet to be completed analysis of the laryngeal behavior associated with 300–500 stutterings produced by approximately 25 adult stutterers. This research is supported in part by a grant from NINCDS to Syracuse University (NS 14351). Stutterers' stuttering, in my opinion, is not as much related to their inability to enter certain speech postures as it is related to their inability to release from these postures and move on to the next sound. Furthermore, I believe that young stutterers' fluency is on a continuum with their disfluency and that these youngsters exhibit the same difficulties with releasing and moving on in their fluent speech, but that this difficulty with releasing during these youngsters' fluency should not be as pronounced in degree as that seen during stuttering. Young stutterers probably begin producing the word-initial or syllable-initial sound with too much physical tension and/or force, but it is their inability, reluctance, or refusal to release, to make the necessary transition onto the next sound, that forces them, if you will, to prolong or reiterate the first sound.

Therapy with these children (as with adults, but using different methods) should focus on three factors: (1) the child's psychological and physiological reaction *just before* he or she speaks (what and how are they getting ready to speak), (2) the child's speech physiological strategy used to *enter* the production of the initial sound of the word, syllable, phrase, or sentence (the child's arresting gesture [McDonald 1964]), and (3) the child's physiological strategy used to *release* from this sound and move on to the next sound. Like a stack of blocks, these three factors support and relate to one another, and the child's inability to release is probably the end-product of a behavioral chain that originated prior to the child's beginning to speak. Such therapy procedures as Van Riper's (1973) "pullout" or Williams' (1971) instruction to "move on" are among the many ways of assisting the child to make the necessary and appropriate releasing and transitional gestures into the next sound. The problem with instructing the child to concentrate on releasing and transitions is (1) they may tend to simply prolong the second sound and (2) speech transitional gestures are difficult to discuss and describe.

One suggestion, if the child understands cursive writing, is to use the transitional written gestures between written symbols as an analogy. That is, the connecting lines between written letters in cursive writing are something like the transitional gestures known to occur in speech production. These connecting lines, the child is told, must be made in smooth and easy fashion for the writer's cursive writing to be fluent. If the writer refuses to, or is reluctant to, or is afraid to, or cannot make the necessary transitional lines between letters, he or she will get stuck on the initial letter. Having the child say his or her name in time to writing may give the child the idea of sound production and movements between sounds. Obviously, going into the word-initial sound with too much physical force or tension will throw everything off. This too may be analogized through the use of writing. Indeed, the child can practice hard and easy writing to get the point that he or she must enter the word-initial sound with appropriate force and tension (not too much or too little) and then must concentrate on smooth, easy release and transition into the next sound. These procedures can give the child the idea of what forward movement in a seriated motor task like speech is all about and also help the child understand what he or she is doing which interferes with that forward movement. As always, the emphasis is on strategies, or plans, or programs, or rules rather than on specific sounds, or syllables, or words that are difficult. The child needs help in understanding that he or she can use the same principle for many different sound-situations. We should try to help children understand that rather than learning one rule for /s/ and another for /t/, they have only to learn one rule for all sounds. The rule to which we refer is that smooth easy movement into the first sound is followed by smooth easy movement into the following sound. There is no doubt that all of this will require concentration and work (we never said any of this would be easy); lasting behavioral change does take time and effort. It is your job to see that the child expends the necessary effort without becoming overwhelmed and discouraged.

Above all, do not turn the child and his or her parents off to speech therapy. Closely monitor the child for signs that he or she is becoming bored, disinterested, unmotivated, and fatigued during your therapy sessions. This is not to say that all therapy sessions should be a rollicking good time or that children and their parents will not have to work hard during therapy and outside of therapy. However, it is also important to maintain the child's enthusiasm for change in speech behavior and a belief that such change is possible. Speech-language pathologists can do harm by providing the child with such an aversive, nonrewarding experience at an early age that it may take many years before the child can forget this experience and be willing to resume therapy. Give children a break from therapy when they or you are becoming stale and apparently bored with the process, but be sure to let the child, parents, classroom teachers, and other important adults in the children's environment know that and why you are doing it. Moreover, be sure to let the child and related adults know the exact time and date when you will resume therapy. Three to six weeks is a good break period, but individual clients' needs will dictate the exact nature of such a break. Homework given during the break should be minimal or nonexistent; let children alone, give them some time to think about whether or not they are interested and willing to make the necessary changes in their speech. Be sure to let parents know that they may call any time they want during the break but that they should not revert back to older, less appropriate ways of correcting the child's speech during the period of therapy rest. Upon children's return to therapy, greet them in as positive a tone as possible, let them know that you are glad to see them once again and that you both can now get down to work on speech. The power of suggestion, as Van Riper aptly points out (1973) and the field of medicine well understands (Benson and McCallie 1979), is tremendous, and the speech and language clinician should use it to help children believe they can change and work toward that goal. Like the little engine, the young child can be helped to believe, "I think I can"; the clinician certainly does not want to add anything to the child's all too common "I think I can't" philosophy. Undoubtedly, the speech and language clinican, as Starbuck (1974) and Prins (1974) discuss, is a motivator as well as a changer of behavior; thus, the clinician must constantly be assessing the child's motivation and must adjust clinical strategy to accommodate the natural rises and falls of client motivation.

○ REFERRALS TO OTHER PROFESSIONALS

It has been said that the trouble with education is that everybody has a little of it. Unfortunately, speech and language suffers from the same problem: Everybody uses it, and therefore everybody understands it, right? Wrong! Many readers of these pages devote their professional lives to an understanding of normal and disordered processes of speech, hearing, and language and yet still feel as if they have an inadequate understanding of these processes. This is not to say that our profession corners the market on information or knowledge regarding speech and language but that our professional training and positions put us in the best situation to deal with the myriad of communication problems that people present.

It is important to realize, however, that certain clients have problems that go beyond our scope of training and jurisdiction or have concomitant problems besides stuttering that warrant attention from other professionals. With children, such professionals are most apt to be classroom teachers, special education teachers, reading specialists, family physicians, the child's pediatrician, child psychologists (and psychiatrists), audiologists, and otolaryngologists. Academic and related matters are often picked up prior to your entrance into the child's life; however, it is not uncommon for certain things like reading problems or fine or gross motor coordination skill to be detected for the first time in an initial speech and language evaluation. The parents should be told, in as nonalarming tones as possible, that such problems are apparent and that you will (with their permission) pass this information on to the appropriate school authorities.

Other situations exist, for example, a child who fails a hearing screening, or who appears to have abnormal reflexes, or who is extremely hyperactive, in which nonschool professionals need to be consulted. Once again, you explain to the parent, in as clear and nonalarming tones as possible, your observations and recommend that the child be given a routine evaluation by the family physician or pediatrician (whichever the parents use and prefer) to assess whether your observations warrant concern. We are not physicians, nor are we psychologists or classroom teachers; neither, we might add, are these professionals speech and language pathologists! While a psychologist might observe and describe what to him or her is a speech problem, it is our purview and professional responsibility, after having the case referred to us by the psychologist, to make the evaluation and diagnosis and therapy recommendations regarding the child's speech and language function. Telling the parents of your observations and allowing the parents to decide if they want further consultation with appropriate personnel is probably the most appropriate route to travel. In a few cases, with parents of limited understanding, you may have to be more insistent and actually make some phone calls yourself, especially if the nature and degree of the problem warrants thorough and immediate attention from a nonspeech and language pathologist professional. As a matter of course, we tell the parents (after they have signed the appropriate parental consent and release form) that we will send to their family physician or pediatrician a copy of our report, findings, and recommendations, unless, of course, they would rather we did not. Although you always run the risk of another professional's misinterpreting, or misunderstanding, or ignoring your report, it is my belief and experience that more information is better than less information and so we continue to send reports to the family's other attending professionals.

In some situations, when the child's problem is not stuttering but psychosocial, a referral to appropriate psychological or psychiatric agencies is in order. Many times, however, the parents and their child may resist such referral and insist that nothing is wrong besides the speech. If you believe, however, that speech disfluency is not a significant problem or that it is secondary to some more serious psychosocial concern (this seems to be the case with about 5 percent to 15 percent of our child and adult stuttering population), then the client and family should be told. And if push comes to shove, and the parents will not take your recommendation, then you have to decline services to the child because you feel it is not appropriate to administer speech therapy for such a problem. It is in your and your clients' best interest for you to develop and cultivate professional interaction with psychologists who work with children and their families; these professionals can many times enter into such tough counselling situations and assist the parents in seeing that psychological services are warranted and most appropriate.

O GENERAL SUGGESTIONS REGARDING PARENT COUNSELLING

Although we have previously discussed the role and manner of counselling with the parents of youngsters who stutter, it is appropriate to recapitulate some of the more salient aspects of this counselling. Cooper

(1979) discusses some of these aspects in very clear and understandable terms, and his booklet should be reviewed to gain some of his insights.* One thing that most authorities seem to agree on at this point is the need not to make parents feel guilty about their child's speech behavior. LeShan (1963) writes about this point at length, and we believe it is important to remember and consider in parent counselling. Instead of engendering feelings of guilt, we, as speech and language pathologists, should try to provide parents with information about speech and language behavior in general and stuttering in specific. We should support parents in their attempts to understand and explore their feelings and their role in their child's general and communicative development. Such exploration may take many meetings with you, depending on the nature and type of parental feelings and concern.

Besides avoiding the development of parental guilt, the speech and language pathologist should recognize the individual nature of each child and parent. Too often, because of the shortness of the clinical day and our many clients, we tend to deal with each parent in fairly similar ways. That is, we tend to gloss over individual differences and try to talk to each parent as though the parent was the typical parent of a stuttering child. This is not inherently evil; indeed, some degree of commonality must exist for our remediation regimen. However, when we routinely counsel each parent in the same manner, we may miss some of the individual parent differences that may make a difference in terms of the child's progress. This came home to me when we noticed a parent telling her son to stop that stuttering! This admonition went on for several weeks during which time the child did become progressively more fluent! Of course, this does not mean that the advice caused the increase in fluency, but neither did the advice cause an increase in stuttering. Perhaps, as Neill (1960) suggests, ". . . it doesn't matter what a parent says to a child as long as the parents' feelings toward that child are correct," and, we might add, the child recognizes the appropriateness of such feelings. The point here is that we frequently give patented responses and recommendations to parents without considering the individual nature, and needs, and concerns of parents. It is the wise clinician who can detect how typical the parents of a young stutterer are and respond both to those aspects of these parents which are typical and those which are unique.

Recognizing the uniqueness of each parent and attempting to avoid increasing parental guilt must be done within the broader construct that these parents are raising children in a highly technical, competitive society. Too often, clinicians, particularly clinicians without sufficient experience, misinterpret a parent's remark that "Johnny can do better in school" or "Sally

---

*Another good source of general information for both parents and clinicians regarding common sense aspects of child raising may be found in Shaefer (1978).

isn't very careful in her work" as meaning the parent is too demanding, perfectionistic, or sets too high standards. I realize that previously I have said that some of the parents of stutterers seem, as Neill (1960) puts it, to "... want to speed up the pace,"[1] but this does not mean that all such parents are overly demanding or that even those parents who are somewhat demanding are necessarily demanding regarding every aspect of their child's behavior. We must recognize the difference between normal parental concern and those concerns which frequently and consistently occur and which seem to be less than desirable in terms of fostering the type of environment where a child's speech fluency can positively develop.

Finally, at the risk of being quite redundant, let me state that parents are people and as the song goes, "people with children." Many of us will eventually become or already are parents, and we should recognize that parents encounter many of the same problems that we speech and language pathologists, as people, encounter. We have tried to carry out our examination of the parents of stutterers within the perspective that we are dealing with people who happen to be parents. We should not be too willing to cast the first stone at parents who, after all, are people like the rest of us, with all our human foibles and fortes.

SUMMARY

Young children who stutter may exhibit varying degrees of the problem. The writer believes that it is not the age of the client that is important, but the age of the problem. Remediating these youngsters' stuttering may involve: (1) environmental modification (information sharing and counseling with parents regarding what they may or may not be doing to facilitate or inhibit their child's speech fluency as well as overall development); (2) speech-language modification (directly identifying and modifying those strategies and aspects of speech production that the child is using which cause the child to disrupt speech fluency, either inappropriately maintain or reiterate an articulatory posture); (3) both (1) and (2) together.

The children and parents who seem most likely to profit from (1), environmental modification, may require some period of time before they show significant progress. It is important that the clinician remember that they have the child for only a fraction of the child's waking hours while the parents spend most of the remaining hours with the child. If environmental issues are apparently contributory to the child's stutterings, they need to be addressed for *long-term* improvement in speech fluency. Children who would seem most likely to benefit from (2), speech-language modification, are children

---

[1] A. Neill, *Summerhill: A Radical Approach to Child Rearing* (New York: Hart Associates, 1960), page 253. Reprinted by permission.

who are prolonging sounds (particularly if these prolongations are silent or inaudible in nature) and generally avoiding eye contact with listener. Directly identifying these youngsters' stutterings and showing them how they produce them and how they may be changed is the best procedure. The third group (3) may be children who fall between the first two or perhaps include many of the second group. Here the child's external and internal "environment" appears to meld to negatively influence the child's speech fluency. The use of real-world analogies, clear, age-appropriate models of the human vocal tract, and audio-visual aids is discussed and recommended.

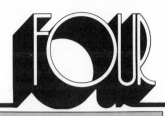

○ INTRODUCTION

○ OLDER CHILDREN WITH MINIMAL OR LITTLE AWARENESS OF STUTTERING

    desensitization

    ignoring the child: a potent but difficult to discern fluency disruptor

○ THE OLDER CHILD DIFFERS FROM THE YOUNGER CHILD

    encouraging the child to (non)verbally interact with peers

    the gradual process of learning or learning about learning

○ OLDER CHILDREN WITH DEFINITE AWARENESS OF STUTTERING

    motivation

    identification

    modification

    parent's role in remediation

    (dis)continuing therapy

    making changes in speech

    encouraging child to talk

    practice

○ TWELVE- TO FOURTEEN-YEAR-OLD STUTTERERS: TURNING THE CORNER INTO ADOLESCENCE

    description

    factors to consider

    when to begin and when not to begin therapy

    objectively changing speech behavior

    motivating client to make speech changes

    practice and/or carryover of change

    difficulties gauging changes in speech

    related concerns: academics, social life, and employment

○ SOME PARTING THOUGHTS

○ SUMMARY

Remediation: older children and teenagers who stutter

○ INTRODUCTION

Older children (those of say nine years and older) and teenagers who stutter differ in more ways than just age from those who are younger. Some times older children have had little formal speech therapy and are thus eager for help; other times the children have had several years of unsuccessful formal speech therapy (which is sometimes only taken twice a week for 15–20 minutes) and are not particularly motivated and interested to receive more. Besides the stuttering problems of these older children, they also present the typical preteen and adolescent concerns unique to their age group. For example, a fourteen-year-old girl who stutters, even one who noticeably and severely stutters, may balk at receiving help for her problem. She may complain that she does not want to seem different from her friends, leave school at unusual hours, or attend special classes not attended by her normally fluent associates. She may even tell you (as children have actually told this author) that she feels like a "retard" by coming to your speech therapy sessions. Understanding the unique problems of the older child and teenager who stutters is crucial for successful remediation.

Parents of these children also have special concerns. Perhaps they have been trying for years to get appropriate assistance for their child but have met with little success. On the other hand, they may have observed their child receive numerous hours of therapy and related services without much appreciable progress. Furthermore, these parents may be having the typical concerns with their rapidly maturing youngster that other parents of children of similar age experience: concerns with schoolwork and academic achievement, dating and relations with the opposite sex, (mis)use of drugs and alcohol, and future employment possibilities. We have mentioned before that the child who stutters and the parent of that child are children and parents first, respectively, and only secondly involved with stuttering. As alluded to previously, stuttering does not develop and operate in a hermetically sealed container but is interwoven with the fiber of human existence. Speech-language pathologists are encouraged to gain understanding of the general human background against which the stuttering foreground exists. We feel that with the child who is older, we become less and less able to separate out our own feelings of how things should be done because the child gets closer to our own age. I feel this dilemma, which is discussed further in the next chapter when we cover adults who stutter, arises because we begin to see with these children and parents, more clearly than with younger children and parents, problems that we ourselves have not successfully coped with in our own personal lives.

Much basic and applied research needs to be funded and undertaken to determine whether the older child and teenager who stutters is different than those children who, at an earlier age, with therapeutic intervention became fluent. That is, does the older child and teenager who stutters present a different situation with more complex problems than does the young stutterer who becomes fluent? Did these older children, for example, take longer to develop reading skills or fine motor control over speech musculature? Were there subtle differences in the home life of these older children which contributed to and perpetuated stuttering? Why is the twelve to fourteen age range sometimes so challenging in terms of successful remediation? These questions and others await empirical investigation for answers. For now, however, there are insights and procedures that we may discuss which have relevance to these clients.

Earlier we said that it is not the age of the client with the problem, but the age of the problem with the client that is important. We were trying to point out how important it is to consider each child in terms of his or her presenting situation, rather than some set rule that such and such an age child should be dealt with so and so. The problem with this sort of approach is that it does not readily lend itself to the confines of an organized book! Thus, for the sake of discussion, we have partitioned our clients who stutter into three age groups: (1) children who stutter, (2) older children and teenagers who stutter, and (3) adults who stutter. This partition is not arbitrary since each age group does appear to have unique aspects and concerns; however, this does not mean that every client in a particular age group (see Table 2–2) will be treated in exactly the same fashion. What we are attempting to emphasize here is that there are some common themes to older children and teenagers who stutter, but that each client presents his or her own variation on these themes. Our job is to learn these themes but to be cognizant and prepared to deal with their variations!

For the purposes of this chapter's discussion, we have divided older children and teenagers who stutter into three different groups: (1) older children with little or marginal awareness of stuttering, (2) older children with definite awareness of stuttering, and (3) teenagers with definite awareness of stuttering. This writer has seen some teenagers with minimal awareness of their stuttering, but these are probably the exception rather than the rule. Further, we have seen a handful of individuals who began their stuttering in their teenage years, but this group is also probably the exception and not the rule. The children and teenagers we discuss have been stuttering for sometime, and the origins of their problem are generally traced back to preschool or early elementary school years. To begin, let us consider older children with apparently little or no awareness of stuttering.

○ OLDER CHILDREN WITH MINIMAL OR LITTLE
AWARENESS OF STUTTERING

Awareness of an event takes at least two different forms: (1) general or (2) specific. The former is predominantly, for the sake of this discussion, an emotional-feeling level of awareness while the latter is an intellectual-cognitive level of awareness. Dichotomizing awareness in this manner is somewhat artificial because most of our awareness of ourselves, our actions, and the world around us involves both intellectual and emotional processes. That is, our intellectual and emotional selves are inextricably related to one another.

On a clinical level, however, it is useful to treat and discuss our clients' awareness of their behavior in terms of objective and subjective components. Many clients of this age group will tell you, in a very emotional manner, that they stutter because they are stutterers (an interesting tautology), but when asked to show or describe what they do that they call stuttering, they will say, "I stutter." Along these same lines, Wingate (1976) has remarked that ". . . it is surprising how poorly most stutterers are acquainted with their own difficulty."[1] We would add that this acquaintance is not as poor on the emotional (general subjective) level as it is on the intellectual level.

When we say that younger or older children who stutter are unaware of their stuttering, we seem to actually be saying that they are not bothered by their speech. A young child of any degree of normal intellectual skills must be aware, on some level, of the fact that he or she talks differently from others. And if the child is not aware, we can be sure that some other, less sensitive, youngster will unsubtly remind him or her of the child's difference and difficulty in talking. Perhaps, then, what we are saying when we say that a child is *unaware* is that the child shows no overt signs of being emotionally concerned about his or her speaking problem. Not being concerned and not being aware are related but different issues. Intuitively we would like to see the child's speaking difficulties diminish prior to the child's becoming concerned about them, but we really cannot assume that the child is not aware of his or her speaking difficulties.

Certainly, as speech-language clinicians, we try to do nothing to increase children's concern, worry, anxiety, or bother about their speaking; thus, we might avoid directly dealing with children's disfluencies and instead, for example, work on speech articulation errors. We submit that it is not the

---

[1]M. Wingate, *Stuttering Theory and Treatment* (New York: Irvington Press, 1976), p. 331. Reprinted by permission.

awareness of a problem that is a problem but the *type* of awareness and whether this awareness generates concern on the part of the child (and parents). If we maintain an objective, matter-of-fact approach to children and their speech behavior, we believe we can circumvent the problem of developing emotional awareness and bother. This, of course, is harder than it sounds, and not all clients will react similarly. We have seen children with no apparent emotionality associated with their speech refuse to listen to themselves on an audio tape recorder or watch themselves in a mirror as they spoke. We have also witnessed children with high levels of emotionality associated with their speech react objectively and positively to the clinician's description of their speaking problem. It is hard to judge in advance, and it is this difficulty which makes speech-language pathologists hesitant in rushing headlong into making such decisions.

Children of nine and older who present physically effortless repetitions are probably aware, on some level, of their speech disfluencies. These children can often be helped through parental counselling, support, and encouragement to continue and enjoy talking. They can be assisted in understanding mistakes in their speech by the examination of mistakes in other activities they or other people they know engage in, like sports, schoolwork, and play. Williams' (1971) *hard* and *easy* speech concept may be used depending on the degree to which the child appears to be moving in the direction of more and more disfluencies. Fostering awareness in this case, as in subsequently discussed cases, begins with those events that do not directly influence or are not produced by the child (for example, how other people make mistakes when they print or write or how the clinician is having troubles learning to ski). As the child begins to understand the concept of mistakes, the gradual nature of learning, and so forth, appropriate awareness can be developed. This awareness is specific and nonemotional; the clinician examines the child's speech and related behavior in intellectual, objective terms. The clinician's noncritical acceptance of the child's speech disfluencies will go a long way towards helping the child deal with these behaviors in objective ways. One caution: speech-language pathologists, like the parents of stutterers, can convey concern and worry through nonverbal as well as verbal means. In fact, the child may actually pay more attention to and learn more from your facial gestures than the specific words you say and use. Too many listeners, when they hear a child, teenager, or adult stutterer stutter, tend to hold their breath, avert eye contact, and immobilize their facial expression. Children, we can be sure, pick up on and react to these nonverbal gestures.

We present this discussion of awareness to call attention to the ambiguities and uncertainties of dealing with awareness of stuttering. Objective awareness would appear to be a positive force for identifying and changing unwanted or inappropriate behavior. Subjective awareness, with its often attendant negative emotionality, is not viewed as a positive force and can contribute to a child's negative reaction to speech. Speech-language pathologists need to know the difference between the two types of awareness and how to increase and decrease both if the need arises.

desensitization

One procedure that we find of assistance with this type of child (and the younger child with an obvious stuttering problem) is a desensitization approach (Hall 1966; Van Riper 1973). In this approach, the clinician attempts to help the child develop more tolerance for events which are associated with or precipitate nonfluency. Because the clinician never actually deals directly with speech modifications or concerns, desensitization is particularly useful with children whose subjective awareness and concern regarding stuttering appears minimal. That is, the clinician is creating and controlling the communication situation in such a way that the child's involvement is that of a spontaneous speaker rather than a modifier of speech behavior. In essence, the speech-language pathologist tries to raise the youngster's tolerance level for *fluency disruptors* for which it seems the child's threshold for frustration is low. Children are systematically presented with stimuli that have greater or lesser abilities to negatively influence their fluency.

To begin, the speech-language pathologist tries to create a communication-emotional situation that is as free as possible from any pressures or frustrations (fluency disruptors) believed to precipitate the child's disfluency. The clinician can gauge the success of this situational control by monitoring the child's speech. When the child's speech is essentially fluent, when the child has reached what is termed a *basal fluency* level, the clinician assumes that she or he has minimized important fluency disruptors. The child's speech at this point should be fluent, and the child should appear to communicate freely and with apparent comfort.

It behooves the clinician to recognize the salient aspects of the situations in which basal fluency occurs because the child may have to be repeatedly brought back to basal fluency during the course of therapy. Once basal fluency can be reliably obtained and maintained for an appropriate period of time relative to the child's severity of problem and stage of therapy, the speech and language pathologist can begin to introduce fluency disruptors or *barbs*. Before going any further, let us state that this form of therapy, as most other forms, relies heavily on the speech-language pathologist's ability to clearly discern what stimuli and events are facilitative and which are inhibitory to fluency. Once again, take children with the fluency disruptors they present rather than those you feel they present or those you are familiar with. Many therapies achieve little success in the clinic, not because they are fundamentally unsound forms of remediation, but because the therapies are poorly applied or poorly understood.

In all fairness, of course, some therapies are poorly stated and thus lead to misapplication in the clinic. The speech-language pathologist must spend some time assessing and testing out which events are fluency disruptors and which events are fluency facilitators and with which children, and when. This assessment is no small task and is just another reason for considering remediation as ongoing diagnosis.

The barbs introduced into the speaking situation are used to toughen children to fluency disrupting influences. Barbs should be selected from events children are likely to encounter in their outside-the-clinic environment. We have used the following events as barbs: answering children's questions with questions; asking questions that involve rather large, abstract responses from children; changing the topic of conversation with children; looking away while children talk; interrupting children while they talk; asking children to repeat themselves; asking children to hurry up their responses. This list is, of course, only partial and is presented solely for the purposes of examples. It is not meant to be all inclusive. On first glance, these fluency disruptors look like "cruel and unusual punishment," but under the right circumstances, done in the right manner (without ever provoking the child's stuttering), they can be used to positively influence the child's fluency and strengthen the child's tolerance for or desensitize the child to such fluency disruptors.

It goes without saying that many children experience such disruptors in their everyday communication situations, and it is only prudent to help them learn how to effectively deal with these disruptors if they are giving signs that they are having difficulty. Each disruptor, or barb, is presented into the speaking situation only until the child indicates that he or she may begin to become disfluent. The speech and language pathologist removes the disruptors *before* the child begins to stutter, not *after*. Much like the medical specialist (allergist) the current writer sees and who treats him for allergies, the allergen dosage used in the desensitization injections we receive is slowly increased but leveled off at any signs that the desensitization shot is precipitating an allergic reaction (sneezing, wheezing, or itching). If need be, the allergist may even back down the level of our allergen dosage, say from 0.3 cc to 0.2 cc, if the higher level causes us too many problems. Likewise, the speech and language pathologist is not trying to elicit stuttering but to slowly and systematically increase the child's ability to react fluently to communicative situations which are increasingly stressful.

Success with this procedure will be relative to the nature of the child and the type and severity of stuttering problem the child presents. For example, fluency during the introduction of fluency disruptors for one child may be 5 percent disfluency or less whereas for another child it may be much closer to 1 percent or less. The clinician uses this procedure to help the child successfully resist the types of fluency disruptors which he or she will encounter during speaking situations. This procedure may or may not be used when the speech-language pathologist is *directly* working on identifying or modifying specific instances of disfluency (its use being determined by the clinician's judgment as to its compatibility with direct modification of speech). The emphasis with this desensitization therapy is one of the situations that evoke disfluency and the child's ability to fluently respond to these situations. It is the child's *tolerance level for fluency disruptors* and *not the disfluencies themselves* which the speech-language pathologist will try to influence. In this case, the disfluencies are a sign of the relative success of the child in coping with the pressures. And as stated before, this form of therapy is ideal for children with a definite stuttering problem but whose subjective-emotional awareness of the problem is very slight. In addition, we like to meet with the child's parents and discuss some of the fluency disruptors they may knowingly or unknowingly be imposing on their child. Along these lines, Zwitman (1978) explicitly describes some parental reactions to children's speech which *do*, (for example, pay attention to *what* the child says) and *do not* (for example, appear angry or impatient) facilitate fluency. The key here is frequency and consistency of occurrence of fluency disruptors because all parents, indeed all listeners, impose fluency disruptors upon the people who talk to them.

Ignoring the child: a potent but difficult to discern fluency disruptor

One sort of subtle fluency disruptor that some parents unwittingly impose on their child is ignoring their child when he or she talks to them. For example, this is seen when the parent and another adult are talking and the parent's child *continually* tries to interrupt to ask the parent something or to get the parent's attention. The child may repeat ten to fifteen times (I've counted!), "Daddy" before the father will respond; sometimes the father may never respond. Instead of the parent stopping the adult conversation and explaining to the child that it is impolite to butt in or telling the child to wait his turn, the parent ignores the child. To my mind, the only thing worse than destructively criticizing someone is not paying any attention at all to the person. Children who must constantly repeat and lobby for their parent's attention experience more than their fair share of fluency disruptors (besides desensitizing the child to these disruptors, we should also try to mitigate their excessive occurrence). Although exasperating, especially after a long day of work, the parent should try to at least let the child know that he or she was heard and that after such and such is done, the child will be listened to. Another example of this is the busy mother preparing dinner over the kitchen counter when her child comes up behind her and starts explaining what the neighbor's dog just did. The mother, as she slices the carrots, says such things as, "Hmmm" or "Oh yeah" while the child rattles on about the canine. Perhaps, the mother does not even say anything but silently nods her head and concentrates on the vegetables. The child, who meanwhile begins to feel she is losing her audience (if she ever had one), gets frustrated and may begin to repeat. Interestingly, *now* the mother turns and reacts either overtly or covertly to this new form of utterance. The message: when you begin to lose your audience, start to repeat; it gets their attention every time! Helping parents recognize (and reduce) and the child resist such fluency disruptors is one of the tasks of the speech-language pathologist. While this desensitization procedure has seen much use with younger children who stutter (Hall 1966), its use with older children is quite appropriate. One cannot claim that the child will success-fully deal with all fluency disruptors and frustrations as a result of this form of therapy, but it is a good beginning, a good way to, as Van Riper (1973) suggests, "toughen up" the child.

○ THE OLDER CHILD DIFFERS FROM THE YOUNGER CHILD

It goes without saying that older children relate to adults in different ways than they did when they were younger. Whereas five year olds gener-ally do what the clinician tells them to do because the clinician is an adult, the clinician finds that with the older child explicit rationale may have to be given for each and every request of the child. Paradoxically, older children may want explanations for adult requests of them but be put off if the explanation is too detailed or stated in language they cannot understand! The speech-language pathologist, to be successful with these children, must recognize their growing independence and assertiveness and be prepared to deal with the associated behaviors.

Likewise, it is important to discuss with the child's parents, school per-sonnel, and others familiar with the child whether the child is socially, psychologically, and academically developing on course. A child who is afraid to speak, who is reluctant to use verbal expression during social and academic situations, is a child who may nonverbally act out to seek peer and adult attention. Speech-language pathologists must be sensitive to these signs and try to get parents and appropriate personnel to intervene to insure that acting out and inappropriate classroom-social behavior does not become a standard operating procedure as the child moves into his or her teen years. We have seen the situation occur where stuttering becomes the least of a child's problems when that child keeps the classroom in a state of mild uproar and the police routinely visiting the house because they suspect the child of the latest piece of neighborhood vandalism.

With the older child who stutters, but who exhibits minimal awareness, we like to continue the emphasis on parent-child activities. Any event that brings the family together is an event that fosters opportunities for positive emotional, intellectual, and communication sharing. Allowing the child to spend week in and week out with minimal adult-child communication besides, "Clean up your room" or "Be quiet, can't you see I'm talking" is counterproductive to successful remediation of the child's fluency problem. For example, a father who enjoys working with tools around the house could be encouraged to explain their use to his son; a mother who enjoys reading could explain her books, in terms the child would understand, to the child. Whatever the specific activity, the child and parent should be encouraged to talk with and relate to one another. Every opportunity should be used to encourage the child to keep talking; that is, the child should not be allowed to become reluctant and afraid to verbally converse with his parents, and other adults, and peers. A child cannot practice speaking if he or she does not talk except during therapy sessions!

encouraging the child to (non)verbally interact with peers

We also like to encourage parents to see what hobbies, sports, or extracurricular activities their child might like to become involved in or would benefit from participating in. It is not uncommon for these older children to come home every day after school and go in their room by themselves or turn on the television until dinner. Certainly these children need time to themselves, but *routine* isolation from peer interaction makes it difficult to develop interpersonal skills. Further, watching television three or more hours every afternoon provides the child with little opportunity to communicate verbally with others (Winn 1977). Children can effectively remain silent while alone in their rooms or when watching television. They should be encouraged to develop the friendship of other children their age; perhaps this will mean, initially, inviting other children over to their house to play. Alternatively an organized team sport like baseball, soccer, or football might be a good way for the child to develop friends and learn appropriate verbal and social interactions (or perhaps more individualized sports like swimming, gymnastics, or tennis). Perhaps lessons at a local school or community center in how to play the guitar, raise tropical fish, or use woodworking tools may help the child get out of the house and interact with new and different people. Needless to say, if mom or dad can get involved in these extra activities, the greater the likelihood that parent and child will socially and communicatively share with one another common experiences. If children learn some skill or sport in which they can take pride and gain the respect of others, so much the better. These rewarding events can only serve to build children's positive regard for themselves. Further, there is no better place for a parent to see how typical his or her child is then by regularly watching the child perform and play with other children of the same age.

the gradual process of learning
or learning about learning

One caution: Some parents, like their children, do not understand the gradual process of learning. That is, these parents seem to think that all one needs to master a particular skill, event, activity, or sport is will power and positive thinking. They seem most reluctant to accept the fact that complex skills, for example, catching baseballs, reading, using a hammer and nails, take months and years to develop and that the first time you sit down at the piano you do not play like Chopin! Parents' impatience with the gradualness of learning is often inculcated into their children. This is most unfortunate because children, by their immaturity, are already impatient with learning! Thus, instead of helping the child learn patience and how to concentrate on small signs of positive improvement, some parents become impatient, discouraged, and push their child to use skills he or she is simply not ready for or has had insufficient opportunity to develop. In these cases, the speech-language pathologist must be patient and continually encourage the parents to accentuate the positive in their child; the speech-language pathologist should support their positive intervention in their child's development. Interestingly, the parents' impatience with their child's skill development is also seen in their relative impatience with their child's progress in speech therapy. Recognizing the existence of such impatience leads the speech-language clinician to be very clear with parents regarding the short- and long-term goals of therapy and how long, in months and years, the speech-language pathologist plans to maintain speech therapy. Parents need and want such time lines and while it may not decrease their impatience, it certainly makes things less ambiguous.

○ OLDER CHILDREN WITH DEFINITE AWARENESS OF STUTTERING

It is difficult to provide a precise age range for these children. They could be as young as seven or eight but are probably at least nine or ten, with a ceiling of approximately twelve. Once the child gets much beyond twelve, adolescent concerns begin to enter the picture and considerably change the remediation and prognosis for improvement. Older children with emotional awareness of stuttering are producing both sound prolongations and sound-syllable repetitions, and glottal fry and breathy voice quality may be associated with both disfluency types. Eye contact, as mentioned by Ainsworth (1977), with listeners may be poor, particularly at moments in time when the child is disfluent. The child will give verbal and nonverbal indications that he or she is psychologically and physiologically tense.

Many people in the child's environment will recognize that this child is stuttering, and the parents and the school system will often be quite concerned.

Bloodstein's (1960a, 1960b, 1961) description of the four phases in the development of stuttering would probably characterize these children as phase three stutterers (chronic; certain situations, words, and sounds more apt to be associated with stuttering; word substitutions and/or circumlocutions; and little or no clear evidence of fear, embarrassment, or avoidance of speaking, and like situations). While, as Bloodstein (1975a) notes, these phases represent an attempt to describe the typical stutterer of a particular age-development level, they may inadequately describe any one individual stutterer. The emotional concern exhibited by these children may be, as Bloodstein suggests, *irritation*, but it can be concern which is more aptly described as *emotional discomfort*, or *anxiety*. Our problem is that we attempt to put categorical labels onto behavior that is continuous in nature and multidimensional. However, it is apparent that these children know they stutter and are concerned about it although probably not to the same degree as teenagers and adults who stutter.

motivation

One of the first things to ascertain in remediating any client, and these clients in particular, is the source of motivation for seeking therapeutic services. The essence of this investigation can be summarized in the following modified analogy: Is the horse being led or is he coming of his own free will and desire to water? Not too many ten year olds will actively seek help (for example, pick up a telephone and call a professional agency), but many of them will at least tell their parents they are concerned about their speech or that they think they should receive therapy. That is, they directly say to their parents that they are concerned about their speech or that they wish their parents would take them to someone who can help them with their speech. Another group of children will say nothing as direct but indicate indirectly that they are concerned and irritated regarding their speech. Still yet another group will express very little, either explicitly or implicitly, that indicates concern. Parents may be the motivating force behind this latter group coming in for therapy services; sometimes it is a concerned physician, social worker, or teacher who makes the referral. Unfortunately, no matter how severe, frequent, or noticeable the stuttering, children with a passive attitude toward their speech will be children who are difficult to help. No matter how badly the parents or teacher desire fluency for the child, if he or she is minimally desirous of expending the necessary effort to change behavior, then prognosis for change is poor. Starbuck (1974) and Prins (1974) discuss these problems and make suggestions for dealing with them.

Identification

Although situations impact these children's stuttering, we have not generally attempted to modify the association between situation and stuttering. For more complete description of situations, developing situational hierarchies, and systematic desensitization, one may read Brutten and Shoemaker (1967). These authors present rationale and therapy for dealing with situational fears and concerns. Instead, when possible, we have the child's parents provide us with a general situational hierarchy, from most to least disfluencies situations, in order to gain some perspective on those events and stimuli associated with the child's stuttering. Further, we believe that concentrating on the child's problem sounds or words is therapy time misspent. This procedure too often leads the child to develop more, rather than less, concerns regarding specific sounds, syllables, or words. I like to have children deal with their speech and disruptions in it using a more general, problem-solving way.

To begin, we use the previously mentioned garden hose analogy (see Figures 3–1 and 3–2) to help children learn something about their speech mechanism. This helps them come to grips with what they do that is facilitating and inhibiting fluency; however, it does it in a rather down-to-earth, understandable fashion. Rather than concentrate on certain sounds or words, we concentrate on *strategies* the child uses (for example, "stopping the air from flowing at the nozzle" or "making sounds hard with the faucet") to interfere with speech. We try to get children to *physically feel* what they do when they stutter. Hearing and seeing are nice and support the physical feelings, but audition and vision are generally *after,* rather than *before* or *during,* the act of stuttering. Children can come to recognize what they do that interferes with speech and contrast this with what they do during fluency. Identifying and recognizing inappropriate strategies used to produce speech are crucial for the child to learn how to modify speech. Children must understand that they can feel and closely imitate these inappropriate strategies and that these strategies can be changed in ways that facilitate fluent speech.

One problem with identifying and recognizing disfluencies is clinician imitation. Imitation, in and of itself, is not inherently bad, but some clinicians do it in such a fashion that the child may feel mocked. This is not a common problem, and many times it is the child's sensitivity towards imitation, rather than the clinician's imitation, which causes the problem. However, the clinician should be aware of such events and try to head them off (in some cases, the child will have to be specifically desensitized to imitational mocking). Another problem in this area, which is more common, is inappropriate emphasis of nonspeech behavior during imitated disfluencies. Here, for example, we may see a clinician showing a child a sound prolongation on the /b/ in the word *boy* by pursing her lips and then quickly and tensely jerking her head forward as she releases the /b/ and moves through the words. That is, the clinician is teaching something in addition to the nature and feel of the disfluency and its physical locus; she is also teaching the child an inappropriate associated behavior. This is readily picked up by the child and comes to be part of the child's disfluency. Clinicians must guard against such unnecessary head and body movements and only imitate that which is necessary to produce the disfluency. If emphasis is necessary, large magnifying glasses, small high-intensity lamps and the like can help the child focus in on the area and behavior of import.

Of course, these children, not unlike many of us, wish that a pill or some passive device were available that would take away their stuttering. This wish is only natural since humans, like electricity, tend to take the path of least resistance. The speech and language pathologist must help children use their mind and sensing powers to intercede between the communication environment and their speech reaction in the presence of that environment. Such intercession obviously takes much work ("we never said this would be easy") and patience on the part of the child and speech and language pathologist. Sometimes we get so involved with identifying and recognizing the child's behavior that we fail to make the next move into modification. That is, the identification phase of therapy is carried on long after it has achieved its desired goals. Moving to modification is something the speech and language pathologist must be doing, in at least small steps, from the initial evaluation onward. Nothing is as motivating as change, even if it is temporary; the clinician must constantly assess the client's ability and willingness to change as well as demonstrate to the client that change is possible.

modification

Modifying a child's speech assumes that the speech and language pathologist knows what changes in speech signify movement in the right direction. That is, the speech-language pathologist must be able to recognize and reward small positive changes in the child's speech if they are to appropriately reinforce and shape (see Shames and Egolf 1976) that child's speech. It is not too difficult to recognize that a decrease in the frequency of a particular within-word disfluency is indicative of positive change. Likewise, it is fairly easy to see that diminution of inappropriate facial gestures or bodily movements during stuttering indicates positive change. However, in the beginning, when changes are less noticeable, what can we use to indicate that our clients are improving? That is, before the client produces noticeable changes what can we use to indicate improvement?

Here, unfortunately, we come up against a blank wall. In the past two decades, our rush to be clinically quantitative, to count and assess behavior within this or that behavioral theory framework, has led us to lose sight of the content of our client's behavior. We can easily set up charts to depict behavior change over time, but we cannot as easily explain to ourselves and others *what* behavior needs to be charted! Fortunately, recent information (for example, Hutchinson 1974; Guitar 1975; Conture, McCall, and Brewer 1977; Freeman and Ushijima 1978; Zimmerman 1980b) is beginning to shed objective light on that which we perceptually evaluate as stuttering. These researchers' findings in addition to my own clinical observations indicate that two of the first things to signify positive change in stuttering are (1) decreases in the duration of within-word disfluencies and (2) a change in the ratio of sound prolongations to part-word repetitions (less sound prolongations and yet more part-word repetitions). We need to look beyond the frequency count of behavior and into the time course and relative predominance of certain behavior.

Duration of instances of stuttering will start to change as children become more and more objectively aware of where and when in the speech utterances they begin to stutter. As they learn more and more about the where and when, they begin to learn more and more about the what that they do which interferes with speech. This level of objective awareness appears to help many children and adults to diminish the duration of their disfluencies. It is my hunch that longer disfluencies are associated with higher levels of muscle activity or tension than shorter disfluencies and that objective awareness of these disfluencies assists children in decreasing the amount of physical tension associated with their disfluencies.

Helping children *directly* decrease the duration of their disfluencies is hard but not impossible. First, the child needs to understand the difference between being physically tense and relaxed and the gradations of physical tension in-between. This is a difficult concept because the vocabulary used to describe physical tension is generally beyond the comprehension of children. Besides, even adults have trouble sensing physical tension in their muscles (perhaps, biofeedback may be of some assistance in this regard; for a critical review of the use of biofeedback with school-age children, see the comments of Guitar, Adams, and Conture [1979]). I try to help children understand the concept of tension by using the Scarecrow and the Tinwoodsman in the *Wizard of Oz* as analogies. Most children have seen or read the *Wizard of Oz* and can readily identify and imitate the floppy, relaxed Scarecrow and the creaky, stiff Tinwoodsman. We explain through word and deed that speech takes some degree of muscle tension, but not as much as the Tinwoodsman or as little as the Scarecrow. We have children throw balls, walk, run, write, or clap their hands with scarecrow versus tinwoodsman muscles. In these ways the idea of (in)appropriate degrees of muscle tonus are imparted to the children.

Next, assuming children understand muscle tension in terms that are clear to them and that they can relate to us, we show them how they can apply muscle tension in various places through the speech mechanism. We employ the garden hose analogy (Figures 3–1 and 3–2) to help the child more readily identify and sense these various locations. With mirrorwork and face-to-face observation, the clinician makes speech hard at the level of the faucet (larynx) or nozzle (lips), and then has the child do the same. Using magnifying glasses and small high-intensity lamps help emphasize the areas that the clinician wants the child to attend to. We demonstrate to children through both word and deed that they can tense and relax various aspects of their speech mechanism and that these states of muscle tension are within their control, that they govern this tension. The child is then given practice in tensing on sounds and relaxing on the same sounds (the specific sounds are not as important as much as the child's recognition and sensing the difference between physical tension and relaxation). We believe that *lasting* change in speech fluency is based on children's objective understanding of what they do that interferes and what they do that facilitates fluency. We are not talking about an understanding on the level of a speech scientist but an objective awareness that is sufficient to serve the child as a basis for modification.

At this point, other therapy procedure may be employed, for example, Van Riper's (1973) well-known cancellation, pull-out, and preparatory set sequence or Webster's (1978) more recent precision fluency shaping, or others. Although the names of various therapies change and philosophies differ in whole or in part, one common element seems to stand out: The time course of the stutterer's speech behavior is changed. Whether it is a change in the initiation of vocal sound pressure over time (not too gradual nor too sudden) or a pulling out in time of the sound following the word-initial stuttering, all modification procedures for stuttering involve, in one way or another, manipulation of the time factor. This, of course, is as it should be since an instance of stuttering takes more time per sound or syllable than it ordinarily should; therefore, an unspoken goal of therapy is to get stutterers to normalize the time course of those sounds they stutter on or at least reduce it.* Our point is that children need to quickly recognize that which they are doing to interfere with stuttering and then change it. At this point in therapy we continually instruct the child to: "move on to the next sound," "change" (reduce the physical tension and move on to the next sound), or "make the sound easy." Such instructions must obviously be repeated, and praise should be offered for small changes in the ability to successfully follow such instructions. If the child appears discouraged, or confused, or is having a great deal of trouble, the therapy task is changed, and this direct work is dropped until later in the session or the next day. I firmly believe that lasting change requires lasting long-term therapy! We may have to prolong this challenging stage of therapy for some time until the child is ready to consistently make these changes.

*Interestingly, some stuttering therapies change stutterers' stuttering by *lengthening* the duration of their sounds and syllables (see Metz, Onufrak, and Ogburn [1979]).

parent's role in remediation

About this time in therapy, when parents see that you are directly working on changing their child's speech, they may ask what they can do at home. Many times we are uncertain what to tell them! That is, our *neutral tone* suggestion to the child to change can become nothing more than, "stop that stuttering" if said by the parents (or us!) with the wrong inflection or as a means to get at the child. We currently feel that the parent should not use the instructions we use, at least in the beginning, because we have so little control over how some of the parents will use these instructions. Outside of the clinic, my tentativeness in this area reflects the fact that we have been hampered by parents who inappropriately use our instructions to the point that when we use them in therapy, they negatively influence the child. Instead, what I like to encourage parents to do is to keep their child talking, to insure that they try to listen to the content of the child's speech, that they not overly request speech from the child on a day when the child is obviously disfluent, and that they reinforce *changes* in the child's speech. The last suggestion is difficult for parents to implement because it requires them to be able to detect changes, just like the speech and language pathologist. This, of course, means training the parents and more work.

Of course, in a public school situation, parental involvement is often very difficult because of facilities, time factors, and school policy, but in a clinic, involvement of parents is not as problematic. As a matter of course in our clinic, all parents of children who stutter must be present and observe during a proportion of their child's therapy sessions. Parents, unless there is an extremely pressing reason, cannot routinely drop off their child at the clinic, go shopping, and then come back in an hour. We want the parent to know what is going on and to be a part of their child's remediation program. We show the parent what we mean by change in their child's speech; we have them observe the child in therapy and point out to them changes their child makes. We tell the parent that spontaneous examples of these changes at home or elsewhere outside the clinic should be praised by the parent: "Boy, Johnny that was a nice change you made there."

We should add that parent observation of therapy, not unlike student observation, must be *guided* to be of any real value. If the clinician does not guide the parents' observation, tell them what to attend to and why, the parents may gain little from the observation other than fatigue! This procedure may require two clinicians, one working with the child and the other with the parent, pointing out therapy strategies, procedure, child behavior, and progress. Two clinicians are obviously not a luxury every clinic or school system can afford. One way around this, if the parent can observe without the child seeing, is for the clinician to arrange in advance with the parent certain signs and codes that the parent is to listen and watch for and then attend to this or that aspect of the child's behavior. Furthermore, at least in the beginning, the parent should not discuss with the child what the parent has observed in therapy. In fact, in the beginning, the parent should not tell the child the parent is watching. If the child directly asks the parents if they are watching therapy, they can say that the clinician discusses what is going on in therapy with them. With time and positive change on the part of children, they will come to realize that their mother and father occasionally watch therapy, but this will not concern them. In fact, we have noticed that this lack of concern closely parallels the children's positive change in their stuttering problems.

(dis)continuing therapy

When children do not change their speech, no matter how hard the clinician works, several things must be considered: (1) Do the individual children really understand how they are interferring with speech and how, when, and where they can change these interferring behaviors? (2) Is the environment counterproductive to the child making significant change in disfluency? We have had parents complain, once a child becomes significantly more fluent, that the child is talking too much and they do not like it! Some of these children revert back to stuttering. (3) Does the child practice outside of the clinic what you do in the clinic? (4) Is the child really ready to put in the time and effort to make the necessary change? and (5) Have you adequately assessed the child's problem and sufficiently geared your therapy to the child's problem and sufficiently geared your therapy to the child's particular needs? These and many more questions arise when change does not occur or when change plateaus and levels off.

Perhaps this is the time for a break from therapy with all the precautions previously mentioned (Chapter Three, pages 63-64) duly taken into consideration. It may also be the time for you to reassess the client's intellectual and social skills; perhaps you are overestimating his or her ability to quickly and clearly follow your therapy plan. It is also possible that the child's social maturity is still not at a level where he or she can independently carry out assignments at home. Perhaps these children get the idea of change in the abstract, but at the moment of stuttering, when things happen rapidly and they are the least objective, they cannot apply what they actually know and can do. Possibly they know those things which will facilitate fluency but will not do them because if they do, they feel, "It will not sound like me." Sometimes lack of change simply comes down to the fact that it takes too much work, too often for the child to maintain fluency; in effect, the child finds that it is easier to stutter.

We continue to encourage and support those children who do seem to be able to change. We have already mentioned the *placebo effect* in therapy; however, rather than reject this out of hand, I think that we should recognize a powerful therapeutic adjunct when we see one. Nothing is to be gained from being reluctant to tell parents and child that they are doing a good job, that you see signs of positive progress, or that this was a good session. We realize that unwarranted touting and praising of a particular therapy approach has given the placebo effect a bad name, but we also recognize that every clinician, either consciously or unconsciously, is involved with its components in their therapy: (1) the beliefs and expectations of the client, (2) the beliefs and expectations of the clinician, and (3) the client and clinician relation (Beecher 1955; Shapiro 1964; Benson and Epstein 1975; Benson and McCallie 1979). We can reinforce and raise children's expectations for change by encouraging and supporting them. Likewise, the parents' feelings that change has taken place can be reinforced and supported; this in turn will help the parents try even harder to change and maintain change in themselves and their child. Nothing succeeds like success, and we can gain much by telling our clients in positive tones when they are making change.

making changes in speech

Not being able to move on from one speech posture to another when one feels stuck in that posture is a frightening feeling for a young or even more mature speaker. It is a sense of helplessness, of being out of control, or of a temporary *white-out* from reality. Physical pressures are felt in the chest, vocal tract, and stomach region. The children are solely occupied with getting the word out, and they will use any means at their disposal to do this. If you will, the ends (getting the word out) justify the means (speech production strategies to complete the word). It is, therefore, unfortunate that at the very moment when change is most important for children to make, they are the least objective regarding what they are doing that interferes with talking. Perhaps we can equate these feelings to those we have if we almost fall off a high ledge but in the nick of time pull ourselves back from the edge. We feel momentarily panicked, frightened, and do something, anything, to keep from falling. If I then ask you, "Tell me what you did when you almost fell off the ledge," it is almost certain that you will have difficulty. Even thinking through the specifics of this fall may make you emotionally uncomfortable. You may even remember the emotion far better than the act of righting yourself. You will probably be even less clear if I say, "What did you do to get yourself in such a situation in the first place?" The antecedents of the near-fall are most likely to be lost in a haze of emotions. The point is that youngsters who are trying to make changes in their speech fluency must quickly and objectively attend to specific physical acts that they are employing during speaking at the very moment in time when they are the least objective regarding their behavior (see Williams [1978] for elaboration on this point). Thus, the emotionality of the moment of stuttering must be brought within some reasonable limits if children are to make the necessary change. I find that success with making changes in speech leads to increased willingness to make changes and a lessening of emotionality. Once children have demonstrated an ability to make the type of change necessary (moving onto the next posture from the posture they are holding or repeating), you may then engage them in spontaneous conversation. Beginning with noticeable, longer instants of disfluency, the clinician instructs the child—in the middle or near the beginning of the disfluency—to change. We often do this by saying, "Now" and pointing at the child. We clearly reward ("Good!") attempts at changing, partial change, or of course, clearly apparent change. Our voice and our finger nod help the child focus on the specifics necessary and, we think, break through the white out of emotionality associated with disfluency.

If the child does not seem to make an attempt at changing upon our instructions, we immediately back up. Does the child know what we mean by change? Can he or she *show* you an easy change on an isolated syllable or word? I do not want the child to spend an entire session being frustrated by his or her inability to make change. We try to assess right then why change is not taking place. Model the type of change you want. Have the child shadow your modelled change immediately after you. The perceptual reality of the change is that it sounds a bit like a fluent pull-out. That is, the child is moving from the stuttering (either prolonged or reiterated speech posture) on the word-initial sound by making the correct articulatory transitions for the next sound. At first, these transitions might appear longer and more gradual in nature than they would ordinarily, but as the child more quickly and precisely recognizes and changes the original nonmoving-on posture, he or she will shorten these articulatory transitions. I do not want the child to end up with speech that sounds like the ends and beginnings of adjacent sounds were elongated like so much stretched taffy but with speech that sounds reasonably fluent. Of course, on a particular day, in a particular speaking situation for a specific sound or word, a deliberately longer moving-on posture might be appropriate because it handles, in the best way possible, a particularly disfluent moment. In the main, however, the child will, with time, make the movement onto the next sound quicker and less gradually.

We try to emphasize to the child that pushing or pulling on the speech posture of the sound they are stuttering on is only causing them to hesitate or stutter even more. For emphasis, we might tell the child that it is as if they were Laurel and Hardy (or some other silly cartoon or comic figure they know) who keep running into a closed door, each time with a little more force and with a longer start. They need to open the door and move on to the next room (speech posture)! "Opening and moving on" is one more relatively graphic way we have of explaining to children what they do when they make their speech postures hard and exhibit an inability to move on to the next posture. We tell them that they can repeatedly kick at the door, each time with a harder and harder kick, or that they can push on it with all their physical might, but they will not go on to the next speech posture until they open up and move on. Most children seem to comprehend such descriptions and act, to greater or lesser degrees, on these recommendations.

encouraging child to talk

We also believe that an important adjunct to therapy with this age group, indeed any age group, is to keep the client talking. Talking should be encouraged and fostered at home as we have mentioned before. Likewise, the child should be encouraged to talk with friends, and in school, and in nontherapy situations like buying items at stores. The well-known clinical practice of having stutterers accompany their clinicians on visits to stores and shops has, as one of its goals, the maintenance and reinforcement of talking. If the child only talks and practices changing his or her talking in the clinic, the child has less than a favorable prognosis for improvement in speech fluency. It is much like practicing to drive only in the driver education classroom and in the school parking lot. Classroom practice is important, but nothing can take the place of actually using the skilled behavior in the forum or situation in which it must be displayed. "Learning by doing" is as at least as important to remediation of stuttering as all of our skillful and supportive in-clinic therapy procedure.

One suggestion to encourage talking on the part of the child was made by Johnson (1961). He encouraged children to read aloud, at first by themselves, then to their mother, father, or friend. His suggestion, which I use with this age group, helps the child practice talking. The parents, after instruction, are encouraged to listen to the child and be uncritical of the child's speech fluency during the reading. The parents are to attend to the content of the reading; children are encouraged to read something they find interesting that can be read in three-to-five page blocks. This activity is not to take a half hour of the parent's or child's time but more like five to ten minutes every day, or at least every other day. It is the act of talking aloud that is to be encouraged, the physical feel of speaking, and the joy of conveying a message to attentive listeners. Fully realizing the relative intolerance of some adults for listening to oral reading, this activity is not to be undertaken by every child and his or her parents. When it is used, the clinician needs to clearly describe the purpose and procedure of this task and to maintain weekly monitoring of its progress.

practice

Getting children to practice that which they demonstrate they can do in the clinic is a major task of the speech and language pathologist. First, the clinician must make the practice exercise something that can be done within a short period of time each day between therapy sessions. Secondly, the child must see or understand some reason why the homework assignment is being given—busywork will seldom get done. Third, we should explain to parents the nature of the practice exercise and its rationale. Parents need to be given positive ways of responding to changes they notice in their child's speech. Fourth, partial or totally uncompleted practice assignments need to be dealt with as they occur and not allowed to become a pattern. Why wasn't the assignment done? Was it too hard? easy? silly? unclear? Does the child have a place and time each day to practice? Is the child sufficiently motivated to change? Are you a sufficient motivator? It should be stated that allowing these assignments to go undone from week to week is poor therapy and sets a poor precedent. Make it clear to the child and parents that change in speech will come but not without time and effort on their part.

Unfortunately, one of the big problems with practice assignments is that they are handed in, so to speak, at the beginning of each therapy session. What more dismal way to start a therapy session than with the child's report, in deed or in words, that he or she forgot, was not interested in, or did not want to do the assignment? Your scolding will not accomplish very much, but neither will neglect accomplish anything. A talk is in order, where you ask questions and listen to the child's answers. Try to impress the child with the need for practice and with its importance to you and the therapy program. Request the child's help in carrying out the assignment. Let children know you trust them to do the right thing, and encourage them to ask questions when your homework assignments are unclear, hard, or meaningless to them. Show them, actually demonstrate the assignment for them before they leave, and tell them you expect so many minutes per day (a short period every day is worth much more than a long period that gets done only one day per week). Help them develop a chart that they can hang up at home that allows them to check off the days and times when they did their homework. Praise them for successfully completed practice assignments; do not just accept the assignments as if they are expected. Let children know you are proud of them and that it is important to you that they have done their assignments successfully and on time. We should not expect dramatic change with such a complex human problem, but we should reward for successive approximations to the final goal: regular successful completion of reasonable practice assignments.

○ TWELVE- TO FOURTEEN-YEAR-OLD STUTTERERS: TURNING THE CORNER INTO ADOLESCENCE

description

Along the road to becoming a relatively organized adult, we all go through a period of relative disorganization called adolescence. This period of personal development begins for some by eleven to twelve years of age and for most, by fourteen years of age. During this period of time, young people begin to find themselves in the throes of physical, social, emotional, and psychological forces and changes over which they have little control. Sometimes one of the last things members of this age group may want to hear and attend to is speech therapy! The mood swings of this period make speech therapy less than a steady course of action. The young person's struggle with independence from parents reminds one of the approach-avoidance conflict previously discussed by Miller (1944) and Sheehan (1958, 1975). One minute teenagers want freedom and disassociation from parents, and the next they are asking for parental advice and support.

Into this whirlpool of human change enters the speech-language pathologist trying to help adolescents become more fluent. These clients present us with a unique challenge in terms of remediation. To start to begin understanding this age group, one might want to read Ginott's (1969) common sense approach to interactions between teenagers and adults. Ginott covers many of the feelings and actions of adolescents, and for this reason alone his book is worth reading. I am a firm believer that we, as speech and language pathologists, must be well grounded in the totality of the children and adults we remediate. Shames and Egolf (1976) put it better when they said, "Stuttering neither develops nor exists in a vacuum. Stuttering is a behavioral response of a living, feeling, reacting individual who is operating in some form of socially interactive system with other people."[2] With teenagers, young teens in particular, it is crucial that the speech and language pathologist knows the general bounds of that system so that he or she can successfully navigate through its pathways.

We have observed that sometimes adolescents do not appear interested in speech therapy. Paradoxically, this disinterest in therapy may relate to the fact that teenagers are becoming acutely aware of their stuttering and this awareness is beginning to become more and more emotional in nature. They may be starting to develop real fear and avoidance of speech and speaking. Their speaking may be making an already challenging age period even more so because they may be reluctant to be outgoing and speak in view of the embarrassment it will cause them. Just when they might want to become one of the gang and impress their friends (particularly those of the opposite sex), they become shy and withdrawn because of fears and concerns regarding speech. The last thing they may want to do is touch, see, feel, and discuss (with a speech-language pathologist) that which is bothering them the most: their speech. Of course, this is exactly what the speech and language pathologist wants them to do: confront the very thing that they fear the most. Along with these concerns goes the fact that so many things are changing for adolescents. They must attend to so many different things that they may feel they have little time left over for attending to or

[2]Pediatric Clinics of North America, "Dysfluency and Stuttering" (Philadelphia: W. B. Saunders Co., 1968), p. 691. Reprinted by permission.

changing of their speech behavior. Perhaps, teenagers may be likened to a beginning juggler with too many clubs to juggle: some of them are going to get dropped and only picked up later on when the juggler becomes more proficient at balancing many things at once. Teenagers need our patience and support, and yet we feel inclined to direct and scold; we may sometimes lose our patience with their apparently flip dismissal of what we consider well thought out therapy plans. Sometimes the best course of action when we face the challenge of remediating adolescents is a break from therapy where client and clinician can separate, regroup forces, and wait for a more advantageous time to resume therapy. Teenagers, however, must be clear that therapy will resume after a period of time when more time and effort on their part can be applied. Our decision to discontinue therapy may not be agreed on by the client and his or her parents, but periods of plateau in behavioral change and relative uncooperativeness in therapy dictate that something should be done. It is not fair to the child nor is it good therapy to prolong the agony of unsuccessful treatment when a break would be a better long-range solution even though the short-term security of weekly therapy ("At least I'm doing something about my speech") is missing.

Specific procedures for speech modification used with this age group are not unlike those used with clients slightly younger or older; however, with the twelve- to fourteen-year-old client, we must apply procedure in some- what different ways. We need to enlist people in the client's environment that the client can relate to, for example, a friendly school guidance coun- selor, a kindly piano teacher, or a supportive mother or father. These people can be asked by the speech and language pathologist to reinforce change outside the clinic, to praise the client's increased amount of talking, and so forth. When sufficiently informed regarding the client's problem and therapy plan, they can help monitor the client's outside-of-clinic progress. Naturally, the speech-language pathologist should find out from the client who these friends might be and the client's personal relation with each of them. The speech-language pathologist should also consult with the client whether the clinician may discuss with the outside person the client's speech problem, therapy plan, and progress. The client's discussion and responses in these matters are very instructive regarding the client's desires to hide his or her problem from friends and relations (for discussion of the *interiorizing* of stuttering see Douglass and Quarrington 1952) and the degree to which he or she is willing to share personal information with friends. Some of the clients may balk at your suggestions, and others will readily agree; however, it is prudent, as well as good therapy, to obey your client's desires concern- ing discussing of personal matters with outside-of-clinic friends.

A twelve- to fourteen-year-old person who has been stuttering since say, four or five years of age probably has a more habituated speech problem than the six year old who has only been stuttering for six to twelve months. This habituation plus the young teen's fundamental flux in development make it a challenge to change speech behavior. Lasting change, I believe, predicates engaging more of the client's intellectual cooperation than his or her emotion in the change process. Interestingly, as Ginott (1969) points out, this comes about by talking to the client in a manner that conveys your understanding of some of the emotional changes and concerns the client has and is going through. It does not mean that the speech-language pathologist becomes a psychoanalyst or psychotherapist, but as a professional, the clinician develops sufficient sensitivity to recognize the adolescent client's particular needs and concerns. While the speech-language pathologist is not directly involved in influencing the child's psychosocial-emotional behavior, the speech-language pathologist should make it clear to the client that he or she appreciates the client's feelings. Understanding the young teen's feelings provides the speech-language pathologist with a broader perspective from which to view the child's communication problem.

Interestingly, little published information exists regarding the specific nature of the teenage stutterer's speech problem; therefore, we decided to remedy this in part by selecting a small but representative group from our clinical population and studying its characteristics. Table 4–1 presents information for fifteen stutterers in the twelve- to fourteen-year-old age range. Note that most are boys, as was true in our sample of younger stutterers (see Table 2–1), and that many are first or only children. Interestingly, two-thirds of these clients report or have clinically demonstrated speech articulation problems. A similar proportion were significantly consistent in the loci of their stuttering moments. Most of these client's (eight out of fifteen) produced part-word repetitions as their most frequent disfluency type with their mean of 16.5 stutterings per 100 words. These facts suggest that persons who are still stuttering at ages twelve to fourteen are in some ways similar to those who resolve their problems, with or without therapy, by, say, nine to twelve but that their stuttering has become more consistent. We need to keep these facts in mind as we plan our remediation programs.

factors to consider

First, are language, articulation, cognitive, or social concerns evident in the clinical picture presented by the person? Significant problems in any of these areas may dictate that the problems, and not stuttering, should be evaluated and remediated initially.

Secondly, what is the client's past track record in terms of speech therapy? For example, did he or she receive three years of public school therapy to no apparent avail? Has this person received two years of articulation therapy only now to be referred to you for stuttering therapy? What role did the parents have in changing clinicians or therapy agencies? We sometimes think that a client's past failure or relative failure was due to poor therapy elsewhere or a misevaluated case. However, many times these fail-

TABLE 4-1

Descriptive Information Regarding a Sample of Older
Children and Teenagers (N = 15) Who Stutter

The clients were selected because of their representativeness of this age group of stutterers whom the current author has evaluated and remediated. Significantly consistent stuttering determinations were based on the Iowa Measure of Stuttering Consistency (Johnson and others 1963). Presence of speech articulatory disorder resulted from either reported histories of three or more sounds in error or actual observation by the present writer of such a disorder; these data relative to articulatory problems are, therefore, considered preliminary and in need of further, more refined and controlled analysis. Iowa Scale for Rating Severity of Stuttering (Johnson and others 1963).

Stutterings per 100 words spoken
    Mean   16.5
    Range   1.0 to 43.0

Stuttering Severity Level
    Mean   3.5
    Range   1.0 to 6.0

Disfluency Type
    Most Frequently Produced by Most Clients: Part-word repetitions (8 of 15 clients)
    Least Frequently Produced by Most Clients: Sound prolongations (7 of 15 clients)

Child's Age at Time of Initial Evaluation
    Mean   13.6 years
    Range   12.2 to 14.8 years

Sex of Child
    Male   14
    Female   1

Child's Position in Family
    First   7/15
    Second   3/15
    Third   3/15
    Fourth   2/15

Presence of Speech Articulation Disorder
                10/15

Significantly Consistent Stuttering
                10/15

ures are also due to the client, his or her particular problem, relatives and/or associates, or some combination of all three. Thus, a child of this age group who is referred to you for evaluation and assistance should be carefully considered, and all such background questions should be asked. If the client's attendance record was poor and you know this for a fact, you should discuss it directly with the client and his or her parents. At the risk of redundancy we cannot help repeating (and slightly change) Santanya's famous remark that those who ignore history (therapy) are destined to repeat it (see Van Riper 1970; Rieber 1977 for an overview of historical perspectives on stuttering therapy).

Third, try to decide whether the presenting problems, for example, withdrawal from social events, reluctance to use the phone or meet new friends, are more related to teenagers' typical "disorganization" or to their stuttering. Realistically, we seldom can make such distinctions, but it helps if we try to give the client every benefit of the doubt so that we do not overly label his or her problems as those *typical* of a stutterer. Our knowledge of typical teenage mood and personality swings and quirks also helps us explain the client to his or her parents! Particularly nowadays, when grandmothers and grandfathers do not live at home and do not routinely provide parents with perspective, parents tend to think that they and their child are the only ones with these problems. You can help if you have some understanding of typical teen concerns and can explain them to the parents. Obviously, we do not want to be too optimistic about this and will want to identify any real problems that exist and need our attention.

Fourth, do not fall into the trap of becoming a buddy, compatriot, groovy friend, or the like; teenagers need and want adult guidance, help, and counsel. This does not mean you become a Marine Corps drill instructor and coldly bark out orders and assignments, but neither must you start denying your adult experience and professional training and start relating like a teenager to the client in therapy. This is easier for older clinicians to avoid than for those in their twenties who most vividly remember their teens, but it is not unusual to see forty year olds act like adolescents themselves in order to better relate to their teenage clients.

Fifth, and finally, make it as apparent as you can to the teenager that you are the guide and he or she is the person who must do the work. Promising quick cures and fantastic changes are what everybody, particularly the uncertain teen, appears to want to hear, but nothing is more debilitating to the client than subsequent reality which indicates they were misled. We explain to these clients and their parents that we are a bit like a person guiding a tour on which the client and parents are about to embark. We facilitate their trip and point out salient aspects for their consideration along the tour, but they are the ones who must do the considering, who must do the walking and touring. It is they who must pay attention to the landmarks we point out and think about what they mean to them. We cannot and will not carry them on our backs. If they refuse to go down trails we think are of importance, we cannot (and will not) force them. We are guides, not magicians: We can point out ways and means for them to change, but we cannot make their problems disappear into thin air. The concept of guide versus magician is not one that makes the client and parent particularly comfortable because it obviously means more work on their part. However, it is said, on our part, in as honest and straightforward fashion as we can muster. I think it is this honesty and directness that convinces and motivates people. We try to show that we believe that the teen, with sufficient guidance, can and will change and that we trust him or her to put out the necessary effort, to spend the needed time, to make these changes. Indeed, we have to trust the teen because if he or she is not going to make these changes, who will?

when to begin and when not to begin therapy

It is best to begin speech therapy with the twelve- to fourteen-year-old stutterers when they begin to show signs of wanting to actively participate in therapy and have reached some degree of emotional, psychological, and social stability. Obviously, every day that these clients continue to stutter makes their stuttering behavior that much more difficult to change, makes it that much more habituated. However, initiating therapy when a member of this age group is clearly not ready is courting clinical failure and frustration. We would prefer that a client actually says to his parents, "Dad, I'd like to get some help with my speech," rather than the clinician and parents deciding for the client that now is the time, whether he is willing or not, to begin remediation. We need to be patient and exhibit trust in the client's ability to recognize when she is ready for speech therapy; this is not to say that some friendly, gentle coaxing might not be of help for a client who is a bit uncertain. Friendly, gentle coaxing, however, is not the same as threatening and browbeating the child into resuming or initiating therapy. Speech therapy that begins when a teenage client is not ready may leave an indelible mark that subsequent clinicians may be unable to remove regardless of the strength of their therapeutic cleanser.

objectively changing speech behavior

For teenagers ready to receive speech therapy, it is important to positively indicate from the beginning that you know that with time and effort on their part change is possible. It is helpful to demonstrate to clients in the first therapy session or two that they are capable of changing their speech, if only temporarily. It also helps if you can make some of your therapy procedure objective and make some of the abstract concepts regarding speech more tangible. For example, an audio tape recorder with a needle deflector VU meter can be used for a variety of clinical purposes. First, you can record the teenager stuttering while speaking or reading and then play back the recorded tape. The VU meter, in this case, can be used to show the client the objective difference in vocal level or intensity between a stuttered and fluent utterance. You should probably practice this a few times by yourself with a previously recorded sample of stuttered speech so that you can readily and quickly discern instances of stuttering and how the needle deflector correlates to these stutterings. As a general rule, during a sound that is stuttered (whether prolonged or repeated), the VU meter indicates low level or minimal vocal intensity level. This may tell us one of a number of things, but our research (Conture, McCall, and Brewer, 1977) suggests two types of laryngeal behavior associated with this low level meter reading: (1) very closely approximated or adducted vocal folds or (2) widely separated or abducted vocal folds. The nature of these laryngeal behaviors need not be discussed with the client, but you can discuss the fact that they become softer when they stutter. Teenagers can be shown the difference between the soft levels associated with stuttering and the more normal or louder levels associated with normally fluent speech. Clients can come to realize that they cause the needle deflector to move up and down, to go high or to stay at the bottom and that they are stopping the forward movement, in one way or another, when they stutter.

Secondly, the needle deflector on the VU meter can be used to help the client understand the idea of moving on to the next sound. For example, clients can be instructed to maintain a tight constriction of their lips during the isolated production of /b/ while watching the VU meter. The VU meter in this case would probably indicate little or very low level vocal intensity. Clients are then told to "open" and "move on" to the next sound, say /i/, while still watching the VU meter. As they open their lips and articulatorily move on, the needle will quickly move from bottom to top, which indicates sudden rise in vocal intensity which they produced by making the appropriate physiological behavior. Once again, clients, through the VU meter, come to see that they influence the way they speak and that they can change, with enough attention and effort on their part, their speech behavior. (Remember during this exercise to try to insure that the client keeps a relatively constant mouth-to-microphone distance!) One caution: instruct teenagers (and adults) that the tape recorder is *only a means* to an end and that it is *not the end.* That is, make it clear that the VU meter is only being used to help them visualize what is going on when they speak, when they change speech behavior, or when they work on using more appropriate means of initiating speech. If clients are not so instructed, they may come to be overly dependent upon the tape recorder or any device used to objectify or feed-back their speech behavior. Periodically, turn the tape recorder off or block their view of the VU meter, and observe whether they can do as well without it. Weaning clients, right from the start, of their need to rely on such instrumental assistance is very important in establishing transitions between in and outside of clinic and developing sufficient carryover of clinical speech.

Third, the tape recorder can be used with teenagers to show them how to make appropriate vocal initiations and transitions. We start with clients watching the VU meter while we demonstrate a very gradual onset of voicing on a vowel like /a/. We point out the relative slowness of onset and the gradualness of the initiation. Some stutterers, in my opinion, exhibit difficulty going from one vocal state, for example, voiced, to another, for example, voiceless (see Metz, Conture, and Caruso 1979). They seem to want to move from one state to another like going from black to white without any shades of gray. They seem to want to hop from sound to sound rather than smoothly making the articulatory transition (the in-between sound) from one sound to the next sound. Stutterers' apparent tendency toward abrupt, almost categorical (discrete state to discrete state), rather than continuum (discrete state-transition-discrete state), forms of physiological speech production is particularly noted during their initiation of speech. It appears that any change, whether voiceless to voiced, voiced to voiceless, voiced to voiced, and so forth, is a site where a stutterer will try to move from one state to another *without* the necessary transition. It is unclear whether the transition is difficult for the stutterer to produce or whether the stutterer has learned this behavior. All we are saying is that the inappropriateness or lack of these transitions need to be emphasized to the client. The client must learn to employ different speech production strategies. One such strategy involves helping the stutterer understand that a word-initial sound can be initiated without abrupt onsets of respiratory, laryngeal, and supraglottal activity. No matter what the real or perceived time pressures in the communicative situation, stutterers can initiate speaking with an appropriate gesture that moves them from the silence of being a listener to the vocalization of a speaker.

Likewise, transitions between sounds can be shown on the tape recorder in such a fashion that teenagers can understand that they must open and move on to become more fluent. The using of cursive writing, as mentioned before, helps them get the idea that whether they are continuing (prolonging) or reiterating (repeating) a speech posture, they must make transitions between letters or sounds for their speech to sound and look smooth. On the tape recorder, the VU meter will look stationary during a prolongation and then make a rapid change up or down as the client moves into the next sound. To emphasize these transitions, the client can be asked to prolong both the first and second sounds of a word but try to make the transition between sounds as quick as possible. The needle will stay relatively still for the prolonged two sounds but make a quick flick up or down during the movement between sounds. Hopefully, with further refinement of such procedures as the laryngograph (Fourcin 1974, 1979; Rothenberg 1979) and other physiological sensing devices, such speech behavior can be shown with greater clarity in a quicker period of time. For now, however, the audio tape recorder can be used for a variety of purposes besides recording speech and listening to the results.

motivating client to make speech changes

Besides helping clients to make the preceding changes in their speech, we must remember to encourage them to make these changes. This is done by praising, positively reinforcing, rewarding, and congratulating them for their attempts at changing their behavior. According to Ginott (1969), it is important with teenagers to emphasize events rather than personalities. If the teen makes a nice change in his speech, let him know, "That was a nice change, Tom" rather than "You've become a good talker."

Emphasize activity and not the actor. Make your praise emphatic, use positive emotional tones in your speech, "That was a *good* change, Tom." He
may not do much but look at you when you say this, but emphatically stated
praise for his acts will help him develop the confidence and willingness to
work at and make change. He should come to value your descriptions of his
behavior. Keep your descriptions and praise focused on his behavior and try
to avoid evaluating him as a person.

If, after several sessions, a teenage client does not make change or does
not seem to be moving in a positive direction, reevaluate your therapy
procedure and whether the client's parents are being sufficiently supportive.
Parents can make or break clinicians' best laid plans, and you should assess
whether your client's parents have a contributing role in the client's lack of
therapy progress. Sometimes these teenage-parent problems are so pervasive and complex that family counselling or individual psychotherapy is the
only alternative. It behooves a speech-language pathologist to recognize
psychosocial problems in the teenage stutterers he or she treats and to make
appropriate referrals. For example, *frequent* reports by the client or her
parents that she cannot sleep or that she does not seem interested in food
should be thoroughly investigated. Referring the client for psychological
services may be warranted if these problems seem frequent and consistent.
Such referrals, we hasten to add, will many times be rejected by the client
and parents. It is therefore important that you only make such referrals after
careful study of the case and the facts. Do not be confused between *your*
discomfort with dealing with a typically taciturn teenager as opposed to a
client whose concerns are other than those which are typical of an adolescent.

practice and/or carryover of change

Once clients exhibit an ability to make change on isolated sounds,
syllables, and words, you should begin to test their ability to make these
changes in more *realistic* speaking situations. As any clinician can tell you,
however, finding such realistic situations is very difficult. Typically, clinicians take their clients around to other individuals in the building where
therapy takes place or into nearby stores or shops. The latter activity, if not
closely monitored, can degenerate into a series of coffee breaks where the
client and clinician come to relate to one another in a most cordial, but
therapeutically nonproductive manner. Phone calls may also be used to help
the client practice changes, but this, too, sometimes becomes difficult if the
clinician shares a phone with others or does not have a phone and must
borrow that of others.

One secret to the realistic speaking situation is advanced planning. Before we take our clients into a store, we plan which ones, what is going to
be purchased or requested, and to whom the client will be talking. It is wise

policy to talk, in advance, to the store employees about what you want to do and when and what you will do. These businesses are generally willing to help as long as it does not take too much of their time and does not interfere with the normal running of their establishment. Prepare them for the client and his or her problem, and insure that the client asks a simple question like, "When do you close?" "How much does this cost?" Be sure to thank them for their cooperation, and you will be welcomed back with other clients. People generally want to do the right thing if only they know how and get a little praise for their efforts.

Besides advance planning, it is wise to make these activities short and to the point. Instead of ten phone calls, three may do, especially if they are well-prepared for and each one is immediately assessed in terms of accuracy and correctness of production. Explain to the client why he or she hesitated on the phrase-initial sound of the phrase, "What time do you close?" Tell him or her specifically, "You went back to your old way of talking: You first took a deep breath and then held it with your tongue pressed hard against the roof of your mouth (or your vocal cords held tightly together, or your two lips pressed together, or some combination of the three)." Explain to the client what is necessary to smoothly initiate that sound or to smoothly make the transition between sounds or both. Praise the client for his or her effort and encourage the client to try again. Obviously, this much *a priori* and *post hoc* planning takes time, but it is time well spent. Do not let the client just go through the motions of talking to strangers over the phone or in stores, but explain to the client when and why he or she was not (or was) successful. (Sometimes it is helpful to role play the situation before it actually occurs.) Once again, concentrate on the event, the behavior, the activity, and not the personality of the client. For the strangers' sake, try to keep their verbal interactions with the client to a minimum. Simple statements that can be answered with either a yes or no response or a short one- to three-word phrase are best. Further, these rather simple, short statements give the client more control over the speaking situation and minimize elaborate discussions on the part of the client and listener. The emphasis here is on the *quality*, rather than the *quantity*, of the client's talking. Smooth initiations of the word-initial sound generally, but not exclusively, are the item of main import. Do not allow the client to be continually unsuccessful with this exercise; back up and reevaluate: Is this too advanced and have we prepared the client sufficiently? Demonstrate for the client what you want done and then encourage him or her to do it.

Personally, we prefer the use of the phone with this exercise since it can be done in the office and allows for brief but realistic communicative situations. Unfortunately, not every clinician has access to a phone, and using the phone costs money. We need to lobby for the use of a phone as part of our professional apparatus; indeed, I would like to see the phone companies develop special, low-budget phone services for the speech-language pathologists that would allow unlimited local phone calls and that provided outlets for the audio tape recording of these calls. The latter might be impossible since it could be construed as an invasion of privacy, but the former could be easily developed and designed for the exclusive use of speech-language pathologists working with teenage and adult stutterers. Making our therapy procedure as similar as possible to that of the outside world makes our chances for successful carryover that much greater. In the next chapter we further discuss the use of phones with adult stutterers and how procedures like the Relaxation Response (Benson 1976) in conjunction with our change-of-speech procedure can be used effectively to help the adult stutterer more successfully use the phone.

difficulties gauging changes in speech

Carryover of inside-clinic change to the everyday world is particularly difficult to gauge. That is, we cannot be sure that the significant increase in fluency we observe in the clinic is similar to that produced outside the clinic because the speaking situations are so different. This is in part the reason for the previously mentioned store and restaurant visits; however, even these visits are a bit artificial because we tag along with the clients when they go into the store or we sit next to them when they use the phone. These are nice approximations, but they are inadequate for the purposes of assessing the client's ability to use changes during everyday communicative stress. This problem is a bit like the one experienced by doctors when they listen to and measure (electrocardiographically) the activity of the heart while the person quietly sits or rests. These tests may indicate a normally functioning heart whereas the same procedures used while the patient is undergoing physical stress may indicate cardiac difficulties. We need the stuttering equivalent of a physician's cardiovascular stress test: How does the stutterer's speech hold up under conditions similar to those the person finds himself or herself speaking in? The Stocker Probe test (Stocker 1976) is a step in the right direction of assessing the stutterer's speech under speaking conditions that approximate everyday speaking situations. The well-known "Job Task/Home Town" procedure (Johnson and others 1963) is another attempt to obtain speech similar to that used outside the clinic. This is a problem which deserves serious attention and one that makes our therapy carryover procedures difficult to assess.

related concerns: academics, social life, and employment

We find numerous references to indicate that for all intents and purposes, stutterers are essentially the same as normally fluent speakers in terms of a variety of emotional, social, psychological, and physiological parameters (see Van Riper 1971; Bloodstein 1975a; Sheehan 1970b). We should remember, however, that these findings are for stutterers as a whole. That is, they hold true for stutterers as a group, but for any one individual stutterer, they may be invalid. Thus, we can expect to see older children and teenagers who may have significant problems in schoolwork, socializing, and so forth. We must be cognizant of these other problems, when they exist, and plan accordingly. Hierarchical arrangements may need to be made whereby concentrated attention to school problems takes priority over speech therapy for stuttering. Parents and their children should not be expected to attend six different professional settings every week. Unfortunately, too often we are less than knowledgeable about these other areas of concern and professional services. Sometimes, of course, most people familiar with the child, including yourself, will decide that the child's stuttering is central to other problems and that with remediation of this problem the others will improve. This is fine and we have seen it happen; however, it is up to you to see that business does not go on as usual with all other professional services—especially if these other professional services all require the client to take an *active* role in changing behavior or learning new skills. The client and parents can only do and be expected to do so much. We need to allow the client some free time to think, day dream, and rest. None of us would try to simultaneously learn golf, tennis, squash, and sailing; and yet we seem to expect similar types of behaviors from children who simultaneously receive speech therapy, reading remediation, special physical education classes, tutoring with math in addition to schoolwork, Little League, Cub Scouts, and tuba lessons!

Employment concerns with the teenage stutterer and parents are many times very serious and need consideration. The two best sources for such services are school guidance counselors or a local rehabilitative counselor. Why, we ask, is a teenager concerned with employment? Generally speaking, the employment concern centers on future, rather than present, employment. You can provide such professionals, for example, the guidance counselor, with the status and prognosis of the teen's speech problem, and he or she in turn can provide you with information regarding the client's (and parent's) employment aspirations. Ideally, you may also receive information regarding the client's abilities to do those things he or she professes to want to do for a future job. You must realize that your voice in these matters may influence other professionals in their decisions, and thus you need to carefully consider the firmness and accuracy of the data from which you draw your conclusions. Whatever the case, avoid getting into employment counselling with the parents and teen in anything other than general terms. Refer to appropriate counsel in these matters, and keep in touch with that counsel and offer information, copies of reports, and the like. Your job is to remediate speech and language and to be cognizant of those events which pertain to this remediation.

In extreme cases, there may be a need for counselling to handle the teen's and parents' reasonable employment aspirations; this counselling may have to take place prior to speech therapy. Of course, when employment aspirations are in line with the client's skills and these aspirations seem to be a prime motivator for the client coming in for speech therapy, it may be appropriate to occasionally mention these aspirations and maintain therapy interest through discussion of how speech change will make these employment goals more or less possible. Under no circumstances, however, should speech-language pathologists say in effect, "You can't expect to become a lawyer if you aren't going to work any harder than that at changing your speech." This is an obvious negative evaluation of the teen's personality and is also probably harassing the client in the same way that his or her parents do. When in doubt, don't!

Sometimes the child or teen who stutters appears to, or is reported to, have psychosocial concerns. For example, one twelve-year old we managed began to act out in class and against his parents. He stuttered quite severely, and it seemed that the only way he could get people to listen to him, to pay him some attention, was to misbehave. His stuttering made little change in therapy, and psychological services were recommended to the parents. They refused such services, insisting his only problem was stuttering. (They were right that it was a problem, but it clearly was not the only problem.) However, they changed their mind when he set fire to his sister's bedroom! Obviously, not all cases are this dramatic or clearcut, but we need to be aware of their occurrence and should be prepared to deal with them. Sometimes, as Robinson (1964) discussed, all these children may need is the companionship and attention of a significant adult; for some this is an older male, and for others an older female, while for others the sex is not as important as the personality and warmth of the adult. Other times we may need to spend considerable time discussing the mocking these children receive from their peers. As we write this, we notice in two recent diagnostic reports we have in front of us that both parents (one set of parents of an 8.5 year old and the other set of an 8.2 year old) mention their concern regarding," . . . the other children's reactions to his speech behavior . . . how these other children's reactions to his stuttering will have a negative influence on him." Such concerns must be dealt with and discussed because they are one major reason these children come to avoid talking to others, avoid situations where they may have to talk with others, and in general withdraw from social interactions. Although such avoidance and withdrawal may be a normal reaction to an abnormal situation, it nevertheless interferes with these youngsters' development. Telling the children and their parents to ignore these taunts and jeers is about as effective as telling you to ignore the negative comments you get from friends and relatives when you have just gotten a new hair style. Instead of ignoring the comments, the child and parents need to (1) understand why certain people make such comments, and (2) how to say something that will defuse the situation and stop the ridicule. Such psychosocial concerns, which are the everyday stock and trade of the speech-language pathologist who remediates stutterers', need to be differentiated from the psychosocial concerns stemming from psychoneurotic problems. To paraphrase an old saying, we need to understand those things we can help with (and change) and those things we cannot and hopefully be able to recognize the difference.

Reading concerns, language delays, and learning disabilities also occur in this population. The latter, learning disabilities, is still an area where much needs to be known and much controversy exists. Let me just state that the learning disability (LD) specialist and yourself, if you both treat the same child, must come to terms with the significant problems of the child and family and decide which needs the most immediate attention. Further, you may have to do much in-service training in this area, discussing the facts of stuttering with the LD specialist. You should also insure that nothing is said to the child and parents that either raises false hopes regarding cures for stuttering or that gives an overly pessimistic or inaccurate picture regarding the problem and its origins. Communication between professions is crucial for both client and the involved clinicians. It can result in a better understanding of each other's profession as well as mutual respect between professions. Other concerns, like reading and language, may also need more immediate attention than stuttering, and it is important for the speech-language pathologist to understand this and set priorities for remediation accordingly. The severity and nature of these problems will dictate, to a large degree, whether they can be treated simultaneously with stuttering or whether one will need to be dealt with before the other.

The child's family doctor or pediatrician, as mentioned before, should at least, if the parents so decide, receive a copy of your initial evaluation, findings, and recommendations. If reevaluations and therapy are planned, it is also wise policy to inform the physician. Although there is always a risk that other professionals may misread, misinterpret, or poorly understand our communications, they can generally tell when another professional knows what they are about and is proceeding in a prudent, cautious manner. Nothing ventured is nothing gained in these matters, and it is a good clinical policy to let the family's main health professional, the doctor, know of your findings and plans for remediation. This is particularly important when you have decided that speech therapy was contraindicated. Furthermore, if the referral comes from the doctor, you are ethically bound to send him or her information regarding your findings (unless, of course, the parents refuse permission).

School personnel are another group of professionals who need to be considered. Many times they see the child as much as the parents do. An experienced school teacher, administrator, guidance counselor, or nurse can often provide you with information and insights that the child and parent cannot. Conversely, some of these personnel may have what we call *long ears* and hear problems when none exists. We have had situations where every year a particular nursery school or public school teacher sends us a child who stutters. This would not mean much except when you realize that the teacher may only have one class of 25 students every year! Highly coincidental we might say, but experience indicates that these individuals might have known or been related to a stutterer when they were younger or that they have extraordinarily high standards for fluent, articulate verbal expression. Phone calls and letters to them explaining the problem of stuttering and what a classroom teacher can do to help should be of assistance. We do not send literature until we feel the individual has some basic understanding of the problem. This is because I believe that observations and readings in new areas of information must be *a priori* guided to be of maximum benefit and the individual must demonstrate a willingness to read and learn. Teachers can become powerful allies to the speech-language pathologist in his or her remediation of a child's or teen's stuttering problem; however, allies, like flowers, must be cultivated and developed. We never said any of this was going to be easy.

○ SOME PARTING THOUGHTS

We have seen that older children and teenagers who stutter present us with a variety of issues to consider in the planning of remediation. The issue of objective versus subjective awareness of stuttering must be dealt with and appreciated for successful remediation to take place. We have seen with this age group that it is particularly important to realize that we not only help and guide people in the changing of their behavior but that we also must motivate them to want to change that behavior. We have discussed impressing client and parents with our role as guide rather than curer, but this must be done in a positive, belief-in-change manner. We have seen that change in speech behavior involves an objective awareness of the specific things the client does that interfere with as well as facilitate fluency. This objective awareness is followed by discussion, demonstration, and practice at opening up and moving on at the word-initial sound or at the transition between sounds. We have tried to show ways to objectify these changes, for example, the tape recorder, and some of the problems we have when we test these changes inside and outside of the clinic.

Most importantly, we have tried to show that it is important to know when to let go; that is, it is professionally correct to terminate therapy when it is obviously going nowhere. Likewise, it is professionally correct not to begin therapy for stuttering with a member of this age group when all the cards are stacked against successful remediation. Finally, we discussed related concerns, for example, reading problems, and knowing when and when not to refer to other professionals. Hopefully, some of these thoughts will help you help others at a point where the problem of stuttering has lingered too long but has not quite settled in for the duration. Anything we can do for these children to reverse as Van Riper (1971) put it, the "morbid growth" of stuttering, is a step in the right direction for them and their families.

Teenagers who stutter exhibit many aspects of the problem common to younger stutterers as well as some traits common to adult stutterers. First, it must be remembered that teenagers who stutter are teenagers (people) first and stutterers second. The period of adolescent disorganization that we all pass through on our way to becoming an adult is no less a factor for stutterers than their normally fluent counterparts. Second, we should try to address the special needs of the teenager who stutters by using age-appropriate language, models, and analogies during therapy and helping the teenager see that it is behavior not personality that we seek to change ("you may stutter but that doesn't make you a bad person"). It is helpful in therapy to engage the teen's intellectual skills for analysis and change their own behavior and attitudes while minimizing evaluations and lectures regarding emotions or feelings; with the teen, it is important to provide a nonjudgmental, supporting therapy environment. Third, we need to understand any events in the teen's everyday life, (for example, chronic failure to make appointments on time, difficulty with schoolwork, lack of opportunities to verbally communicate at home, school, or with friends) that may have untoward influence on the teen's progress through speech-language therapy. We may not be able, at least at first, to influence these everyday events but we should be aware of their presence and potential contribution to therapy progress.

Parents' roles in the remediating of a teenage stutterer may be minimal, moderate, or considerable, pending the client's individualistic circumstances. However, parents' impact on the teenager, it is probably fair to say, is probably less than it is with the younger stutterer. Remediating the teenager may be somewhat more of a challenge than with younger children but the rewards are every bit as satisfying to both client and clinician.

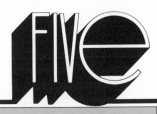

○ INTRODUCTION

○ PROBLEM DICTATES
  PROCEDURE

○ GROUP AND/OR INDIVIDUAL
  THERAPY

○ INDIVIDUAL THERAPY WITH
  ADULTS WHO STUTTER:
  FIRST IMPRESSIONS

  after first impressions

  identification

  I'm beginning to stutter more

  the bridge between
  identification and
  modification

  if identification fails to
  develop

  modification: beginning
  considerations

  modification: where and what
  to begin changing

  modification: after then
  during the instance of
  stuttering

  modification: when the client
  fails to change

  modification: when the client
  produces real change

○ WITHIN-THERAPY
  CARRYOVER

○ CHANGING SPEECH IN
  CONVERSATION

○ HOMEWORK WITH ADULTS
  WHO STUTTER

○ SPEECH SHOULD BE
  AUTOMATIC OR WHY DO I
  HAVE TO THINK ABOUT IT
  ALL THE TIME?

○ WHEN TO DISMISS

○ FOLLOW-UP THERAPY
  SESSIONS

○ SOME PARTING THOUGHTS

○ SUMMARY

Remediation:
adults who stutter

○ INTRODUCTION

An individual who is still stuttering in the latter years of high school and beyond qualifies as an *adult stutterer*. Most often these individuals will have previously received unsuccessful speech and language therapy in addition to other forms of remediation, for example, hypnotherapy, psychotherapy, or specialized academic or vocational counselling. On rare occasions, however, you may be the first professional who evaluates and remediates an adult who stutters, but these adults are the exception rather than the rule. Naturally, a history of past therapy in the presence of continued stuttering means that the adult client may have doubts regarding your ability to help at this point. These doubts, whether explicitly or implicitly expressed, may threaten the speech-language pathologist, especially when many such professionals have their own self-doubts regarding their ability to help adults who stutter.

In addition to the doubts are the client's relatively habituated attitudes, speech behaviors, and beliefs relating to stuttering in specific and speech in general. Such habituation implies that these aspects will be fairly resistant to change because adults who stutter, like all adults, spend many years developing their own personal behavior. They are most comfortable with this behavior because it is what they know best and routinely perform. Whether an adult stutterer's speech behavior is appropriate or not, it is the behavior that the adult stutterer produces and it is this behavior that feels, looks, and sounds most like him or her. This is the behavior that seems most natural. Perhaps the naturalness of and familiarity with the behavior is why the adult client presents the clinician with something of a Catch-22 situation: Clients may ask the clinician to stop their stuttering but they do not as readily request that the clinician help change their means of speaking, reacting, feeling, or thinking!

The possible doubts and resistance to change may also be coupled with rather high levels of emotionality concerning the problem. Indeed, for many listeners, it is the adult stutterer's apparent emotionality, this nervousness, or lack of self-confidence, or unsure-of-oneself quality that is the hallmark of adults who stutter. We cannot count the number of times we have been told by well-intended (non)professionals outside (as well as inside) the field of communicative disorders that such and such an adult stutterer "just needs to get more self-confidence (or less nervous) and then he won't stutter." While there may be some truth in this advice, it is obviously an overly simplistic solution to an extremely complex problem. We believe that the emotionality of the adult who stutters is something that should be dealt with by the speech and language pathologist; however, too many times this dealing is either nonexistent, superficial, or too far beyond the bounds of the speech and language pathologist's training and experience.

Finally, after the doubts, relative resistance to change, and high levels of emotionality, we may also find that the adult stutterer is someone who, on one level or another, is discouraged. Adult stutterers may be discouraged that they do not talk like others, that they may never talk like others, or that they are different from their friends and associates. Like their doubts regarding your ability to help, their discouragement with themselves and their behavior must be mitigated if therapy is to stand a chance of being successful.

Thus, we approach the adult who stutters with caution but with optimism as well. We know that we can help adults who stutter, but we also know that this is no easy task where success will come quickly. The therapy will require constant review on our part and an ever-watchful eye on those aspects of therapy we should terminate and those aspects we need to introduce. If we can begin by knowing what we know as well as those things we still do not know, we have a good likelihood of helping the adult who stutters. We realize, of course, that the adult problem with stuttering differs in both degree and kind from that we have observed with younger stutterers. And we also know that these differences in the problem create differences in our procedure because the clinical problem generally dictates the clinical procedure.

○ PROBLEM DICTATES PROCEDURE

In Chapter Two we covered the diagnosis and evaluation of stutterers and stutterings and do not intend in this space to reiterate this coverage; however, there are a few nuances to the evaluation of adult stutterers that should be mentioned prior to the description of remediation. It should be recalled that stuttering is a disorder of childhood (Beech and Fransella 1968); that is, it has its origins in the developing child. Thus, adults who tell you that their stuttering just began last year when they were a senior in high school, after they got married, and so forth, are adults who do not have what we would consider a run-of-the-mill stuttering problem. These clients need careful assessment, a second opinion from another qualified speech and language pathologist, and perhaps a routine medical or psychological evaluation. We have sometimes been fools who have rushed into places where angels fear to tread, but fortunately we have learned some things from these imprudent moves. One of the things we have learned is to be cautious, careful, and deliberate with regard to remediating stutterers whose stuttering begins in adulthood.

A similar but different issue relates to the overlap in the adult population between stuttering, organic-neurological, and psychosocial problems. That is, some stutterings have organic-neurological or psychosocial origins and do not fall into the category of problem (stuttering) that this book deals with. For instance, some adults with certain types of apraxic disorders (see Darley, Aronson, and Brown 1975) or organic brain damage (Rosenbek and others 1978) have stutteringlike behavior, but this does not mean that they are stutterers. Likewise, some individuals have deep-seated psychoemotional problems which appear to relate to their speech hesitations. Dealing with these two classes of individuals, stutterers with either psychoemotional or organic-neurological etiology, as if they are typical stutterers does not appear good policy. Indeed, the ability to know when and how to refer these individuals to appropriate agencies or professionals is a skill worthy of development.

Lastly, some adults who stutter may be referred to us by their employers. That is, an up-and-coming young salesperson who stutters may be told, indirectly or directly, by the employer that advancement will be determined by improvement in the salesperson's fluency. After discussing this situation with the client and point blank asking the client if we can discuss this situation with the employer, we ask the client to have the employer call us. When we receive the call, we discuss with the employer his or her perceptions of the client and the client's problem(s). In this conversation we are able to impart to the employer basic information regarding stuttering and see how receptive he or she is to such information. We promise no rose gardens, but we do tell the employer that we are positively supportive of clients in their attempts to assist themselves. We try to determine how realistic, supportive, and understanding the employer is with regard to the client and the client's problem. In some cases, we have referred the client elsewhere or declined services because we thought that the situation was untenable in terms of successful therapeutic outcome. Obviously, the door to the clinic remains open to this client, but I explain that given present conditions, therapy elsewhere or at a later date would seem most appropriate.

○ GROUP AND/OR INDIVIDUAL THERAPY

In recent years, with the emphasis on behavioral modification and structured individual therapy sessions, it seems that there has been a movement away from group therapy with adult stutterers. We believe that this is unfortunate because group therapy for adults who stutter can be a positive experience. In these groups, adults who stutter can share experiences and feelings with others who share the same concerns. The group provides a sheltering atmosphere whereby adult stutterers can say what they want to about their problems and others will at least listen, even if they do not always agree! Through a group adult stutterers come to learn that they are not alone in the world with this problem, that others share their troubles and feel much the same way they do. Groups provide speaking outlets for people who might otherwise go literally for days or weeks without talking to other nonprofessionals. Conducting group therapy for adult stutterers is no easy task. The disorder itself interferes with the basic medium of group therapy: talking. If it were easy for stutterers to talk, they would not be coming to you for therapy in the first place! Thus, for the leader of the group, there are periods of discouragement when it appears no one wants to contribute or talk. In fact, many adults who stutter seem to want nothing to do with group therapy. They appear reluctant to even see or hear another stutterer; the reasons for this reluctance vary with each client. The following is but a partial listing of reasons: (1) some seem reticent to see themselves in others; that is, they realize that the stuttering problems of others mirror their own problem, and they resist having to face this reality; (2) they seem to believe that by hearing and seeing others who stutter that they will get worse or stutter more; and (3) they appear to believe that by seeing and hearing others stutter they may catch or pick up more stuttering. Actually, (3) is just another way clients state (2).

We have reached a point in our experience whereby we request that all adult stutterers attend weekly group sessions (unless for an exceptional reason, for example, the client speaks English as a second language and thus the group situation would be extremely difficult for him or her to understand). Attendance in our group permits us to monitor adults' progress in individual therapy and the specific nature of their speech and related problems. We have found through experience that the ideal group size is about seven people, but we have had as many as twelve or thirteen and as few as three. The time is fixed throughout the year, and it generally takes place in late afternoon or evening. We have also found that an odd block of time, say one hour and fifteen minutes, allows people to arrive late and leave early but still get in about 30–45 minutes of group therapy. A one-hour session, on the other hand, is seemingly harder for people to make, and clinicians wind up with too many people coming and going in twenty minutes or less. I therefore like to begin at 3:30 p.m. and end at 4:45 p.m.

If it is possible to arrange, groups of adults who stutter should be composed of a mix of individuals, for example, college students, laborers, executives, and secretaries. In this way you, as well as your clients, learn how stuttering cuts across all walks of life and how it influences different people in different and similar ways. Such variety also insures that students-in-training, if you work in such a setting, get experience observing and managing different individuals. This is a much more realistic experience and preparation for their professional careers after graduation.

An adult client can also receive group therapy and nothing else. This is particularly true for the marginally disfluent adult stutterer whose concerns about his or her speech do not seem warranted by the nature or severity of the presenting speech problem. These individuals quickly see that the nature and severity of their stuttering is far different and considerably less than that of others. Sometimes the most patient, clear presentation of a speech-language pathologist cannot convince them of this fact as quickly as an hour spent interacting with three or four moderate-to-severe stutterers! Thus minimally disfluent clients also benefit from learning that some of their communication concerns are shared by others but that objectively they have less reason for concern. Also, subtle, as well as not so subtle, group pressures ("Why are you in the group, you don't stutter?") influence minimally disfluent speakers to reconsider their concerns, to think about their problems. And, after all, getting our clients to think and change behavior is what it is all about anyway.

None of the preceding, however, should be taken to mean that group therapy with adults who stutter is a panacea. Obviously it is not because the same problems with tardiness, attendance, and failure to do homework assignments that plague individual therapy bedevil group therapy. The group leader must be a motivator as well as an organizer. At times this leader must be rather authoritative in manner and at others very much laissez faire. Indeed, the group leader is the common thread that runs from one year to the next, the person who provides continuity to the group as clients fade in and out. He or she must be sufficiently structured to get and keep each group going but be prepared to backtrack and discard all such structured plans if group behavior so dictates. The group leader must tread a thin line between working on, what clients call, *the mechanics of speech* and their feelings about themselves and their speech. With too much discussion of attitudes, beliefs, and feelings, some clients in the group lose interest and think the group is becoming too esoteric and nonsubstantive. On the other hand, when there is too much discussion of this or that client's or all clients' speech mechanics, some clients may feel that we are slighting their personal beliefs, feelings, and attitudes. An adult who stutters, as I have been told by many such people, is "more than just a mouth, larynx, and speech . . . I'm also a person who feels." Thus, the group leader is constantly shifting within as well as between group sessions from discussions of attitudes to discussions of speech behavior, and back again. Group therapy is, therefore, no situation for the professional who finds it difficult to juggle more than two balls at once! We are convinced, however, that such groups are beneficial to the client and clinician and should be given serious consideration in the development of a therapy program for adult stutterers.

○ INDIVIDUAL THERAPY WITH ADULTS WHO STUTTER: FIRST IMPRESSIONS

We have mentioned before the impact of first impressions on the young children and parents we deal with in therapy. Similar impressions are given to adults who stutter, but the means by which the impressions are made differ with these clients. Obviously, our attempts to convey positive first impressions to the adult stutterers should not be a show or a forced procedure; adult clients can easily detect a show of insincerity. Instead, our understanding of stuttering in general, and the adult's problem in specific, must be apparent to the client from the beginning. Our ability to listen to the adult and our ability to help (without overly exaggerating this ability) is also of importance to the adult. We can give signs of support and the belief that therapy will be of assistance, and yet we should make it clear to the client if we are guarded in our belief concerning the client's prognosis for positive change in speaking and related attitudes, beliefs, and feelings. Demonstrating to the adult client that his or her speech can be changed, even through an artificial means, for example, metronome, choral reading, or whispering, can be used to show that (1) the client's speech disfluency is malleable; (2) that fluency, given certain circumstances, is obtainable; and (3) that you, as a professional speech and language pathologist, can assist him or her in the modification of speech. We use the orientation of *helping with* the problem rather than *curing of* the problem. Once again, clearly and repeatedly, explain to the client that such artificial means of achievement are just that and will not be the principle means by which we will assist him or her change speech and related behavior. We say that it is simply a means to demonstrate change and our ability to help that client make such change. Leading the client to dream the impossible dream that we can cure him or her of stuttering (while the adult stutterer passively stands around and watches), is, in my mind, the ultimate cruelty because time will show that such a dream cannot be realized. The short-term gain of wowing the client with clinical legerdemain is always counterbalanced by the long-term pain of reality. As we point out in the next chapter, quick but total and permanent cures for complex human behavior disorders are not compatible with the present state of the human condition. In short, we want to lead the client from the first meeting into a positive therapy atmosphere where change is possible and desirable rather than misleading the client that we are able to change lead into gold!

after first impressions

Assuming the client agrees and we think it appropriate, the client begins therapy. The first question we ask is: How often and how long? This is no easy question to answer, but hopefully we have told the client in the initial evaluation (see Chapter Two) the approximate time line of the therapy. We must then square the ideal with the real: Therapy every day may be best, but our clinical program and the demands on our time may only permit one hour per week. We recognize that the intensity and/or frequency of speech therapy (see Gregory 1978) may be of primary positive significance to our client's improvement; however, while my experience at this point cannot rival the breadth and depth of some workers in the field, it does suggest to me that lasting, long-term change of stuttering and related matters may take much longer than we or our clients would like. This is especially true, we think, for adult stutterers. Presently, given the time and space considerations of our clinical situation, we remediate adult stutterers on a once- or twice-a-week basis, and the usual time frame (start to end) runs from three to twelve months.

Before we begin such a protracted therapy regimen, we inform our clients that we plan to initiate what I call *trial therapy*. With adults this trial usually lasts from three to six weeks. We inform the client of the beginning and end of this trial and that a judgment will be made somewhere between the middle and end of this period regarding the continuation of therapy. We emphasize that the client does not have to produce total change for continuation, but it must be apparent that change seems possible or that the client is moving in the right direction. We stress the positive but inform clients that before they or we get involved in an extensive therapy program, it must be apparent that the situation warrants the necessary time and effort. It is not unusual in these situations for clients to want to hurry up and get therapy whether or not they are ready and willing to expend the time and effort. You must not be stampeded into these untenable therapy situations. Conversely, you should try to recognize a client's sincere and honest desire to commit the necessary personal resources to obtain the type of desired therapy outcome. It is not easy to recognize the difference between sincere motivation and mere expediency, but it is something we need to develop.

Assuming, for the sake of continuing this discussion, that the client makes the necessary effort and commitment and that we believe we can assist him or her in modification of stuttering, we begin in earnest. The first step, not unlike what we do with older children and teenagers, is to assist the client in quickly and accurately identifying the instances of stuttering. The emphasis here, as elsewhere, is on the inappropriate *strategies* and *behaviors* the client employs to interfere with fluent speech. The problem lies in the strategies the client employs and not in the sounds and syllables the client produces.

Identification

We firmly believe that it is difficult to achieve *lasting* change in stuttering if stutterers cannot quickly and correctly identify when they are stuttering. Unless they can do this, we think that it is difficult to lastingly change stuttering. That is, how can individuals change stuttering when they cannot identify when and how they stutter (interfere with speaking)? Many seem to try, but the *long-term* success of these trials is not overwhelming. Indeed, one of the first things we find out in the previously mentioned trial therapy period is whether or not the client is ready, willing, and able to identify instances of stuttering and if so, how accurately this can be done.

Items to use in this stage of therapy include an audio tape recorder, an audio-videotape recorder (with associated monitor), magnifying glass, mirrors, language master type tape recorder and/or player, oscilloscope (signal generated by microphone fed to scope), flashlight with push-button on-off switch, clicker (like those used by children around Halloween), or any other device that quickly and clearly provides a visual or auditory stimulus for the client's observation. These items can be used in a variety of ways. For example, the client and clinician each employ flashlights or penlights, with on-off push buttons, with the object of seeing who—the client or clinician —can push the button first when an instance of stuttering occurs. As mentioned earlier, it is not easy to get individuals who stutter, particularly adults with a long history of the problem, to listen and view themselves on tape. This is no small concern and must be, with some adults, approached with sensitivity and concern for the client's feelings. On the other hand, no one ever said this process was going to be easy for the client, and some degree of emotionality and self-recrimination must take place in order for therapy to move forward. Likewise, some clients do not react favorably to clickers and flashlights used to "highlight" stuttering (see Siegel 1970). Adult stutterers may say that this procedure makes them nervous, or feel hurried, or statements to the effect that this aspect of identification makes them feel uncomfortable. These feelings must be discussed, and you should indicate your understanding of their validity. That is, do not ignore these reactions, but discuss their nature and their possible causes. Explain your appreciation for the unpleasantness of such emotions. ("I realize that hearing this clicker every time you stutter is frustrating, but this is one way I have of helping you help yourself"). In the beginning do not use these procedures for extended periods of time (fifteen to twenty minutes at a stretch); instead, break them up into smaller blocks of say three to five minutes with a few minutes rest in between to discuss the reasons for success or failure. You can gradually increase the time of identification exercises as clients get more and more adept at recognizing instances of stuttering, as they begin to beat you at identifying the occurrence of a stuttering, or as they are consistently identifying during the middle or towards the start of an instance of stuttering. By no means, however, devote an entire session to identification. Mix it up with discussion of group therapy events. If group therapy is not part of your adult client's regimen, then mention success outside of the clinic, identifying situations that are becoming easier to speak in or relatives' or associates' reactions to the client's therapy progress. Whatever, mix up the content of this therapy hour to avoid boredom and also because identification of instances of stuttering is hard, intense work, and extensive immersion in this procedure is in the long run counterproductive.

We may begin identification in earnest once clients demonstrate a willingness to see, hear, and feel their instances of stuttering (this demonstration need not be one of absolute but of relative willingness). It should be stressed that it is not only important that you know why you employ identification but that your adult client also realizes its importance and rationale. Obviously, identifying something is not the same as changing that thing; however, changing something presupposes the changers can identify what they are changing! The accuracy and speed with which such identification is made is critical. Also crucial, I might add, is the *mode* of identification (vision versus audition versus feeling of physical tension and movement). To begin, we emphasize the accuracy and objectivity of the identification, and then proceed to the speed, and finally stress the mode (feelings of physical tension, movement, and positions).

Accuracy of identification of instances of stuttering has been covered in other sources (for example, Van Riper 1973, 1974). Basically, adult stutterers are given an opportunity to observe themselves during speech and are then asked to label through voice or gesture each and every time they perceive a stuttering. This opportunity can be made available through audio or audio-video recordings or the client's speech productions (*off-line* analysis) or during the actual speech production itself (*on-line* analysis). Off-line analysis, albeit the stutterer's initial reactions may be negative, is the best and easiest place to begin. After accuracy of identification during off-line analysis is 80 percent or greater, the clinician can proceed to on-line identification. However, most clients have difficulty, at least in the beginning, monitoring their speech productions simultaneously with carrying on a lucid conversation. We might add that clinicians have the same difficulty simultaneously identifying instances of stuttering in the client's speech while at the same time trying to maintain normal conversation with the client. This parallel processing (simultaneously monitoring speech production and maintaining cogent conversation) is a necessary skill the clinician must develop as well as to try to help his or her client develop.

Off-line identification. Off-line analysis is best done when the speech-language clinician is *a priori* aware of all instances of stuttering contained within the recording. One way to begin such off-line analysis is to present to your client a previous recording of another adult stutterer who frequently exhibits various kinds of stutterings. The clinician can analyze this recording in advance and even type up a transcript of the recording. In this way, the client can begin to listen to recorded instances of stuttering produced by another stutterer personally involved with the problem. The client's objectivity may be enhanced; at the same time the client gains experience being a constructively critical listener and observer. The typed manuscript permits client and clinician to easily compare notes and go back into the taped conversation at precise points. Tape counter numbers should be tabulated every ten words or so on the manuscript to enhance the clinician's ability to readily go back and forth through the tape recording, instead of wasting time guessing where a particular section of the recording lies on the tape. Furthermore, and most importantly, the clinician's *a priori* listening, analyzing, and tabulating the number and type of stutterings of the recording means that she or he can devote full time and attention to the present client's ability to accurately identify and label instances of stuttering. Too often, the clinician spends precious time in these initial therapy sessions off-line assessing and/or identifying instances of stuttering and thus cannot pay as close attention as need be to the client's difficulties with this task.

We should note that it is important that the client recognize the type of stuttering (for example, sound prolongation versus sound-syllable repetition) as well as the number of stutterings. That is, does the client easily and accurately identify all sound-syllable repetitions but apparently miss many sound prolongations? Similarly, does the client identify stutterings of 1.0 seconds and longer but miss the shorter stutterings, say 0.5 to 1.0 seconds (shorter stutterings than this exist but the beginning client, at least, cannot be expected to readily identify such brief stutterings). These problems need to be discussed with the client as well as the reason(s) for such successes and failures and exactly what the client calls stuttering in himself or herself and others. In essence, the client's relative skill as an identifier of stutterings should be discussed thoroughly before embarking on more identification procedures. The client must be clear on the purpose of these procedures; here, as elsewhere, redundancy of instruction will be necessary. Obviously, your goals are other than merely accurate and quick identification, but the client should realize this because you have made this fact explicit. The client must be clear that learning is a gradual process and the identification step is but one point along the gradual learning curve that leads the client from stuttering to being normally fluent.

On-line identification. After this initial exposure to off-line analysis, the client can begin observing and analyzing his or her own stutterings. The clinician is again cautioned to encourage the client for any and all approximations to accurate identification. That is, the client will not immediately be 100 percent successful in the accurate identification of instances of stuttering (as well as normal nonfluencies), and the client's clinician should realize this and reinforce accordingly. Demonstrate to the client that you understand the difficulty of the task and that you appreciate the client's attempts. Depending on the frequency and types of stuttering, the clinician may be able to clearly target this phase of the identification procedure. That is, the clinician may be able to target for the client the specific types of stutterings (long versus short, sound prolongations versus sound-syllable repetition) he or she wants the client to attend to and identify. As a general rule, it is good to begin with longer sound-syllable repetitions, but if sound prolongations predominate, then longer rather than shorter instances are best to start this phase of identification with. Remember that (1) many sounds are produced per second (possibly as many as fourteen sounds per second [Darley, Aronson, Brown 1975]) and (2) it takes the unsophisticated listener, like your client in the beginning of therapy, a while to decide and identify instances of stuttering. Thus, give the client a break, and target longer instances of stuttering to begin with, so that he or she has that little bit of extra time necessary to make accurate decisions. With experience the adult stutterer will be able to perceive the shorter and shorter instances of disfluency until with practice, he or she can perceive very short instances of stuttering that occur around a reaction time of 250 msec or less. It is time to move on, however, when the client demonstrates relatively accurate identification of most medium-to-long instances of stuttering from a tape recorded sample of his or her speech. We are ready to go to the bridge between off-line and on-line analysis. This *bridge* involves using an audio tape recorder or an audio-video tape recorder that has a pause or instantaneous stop switch or button on it.

The object of this bridge is the *speed* of identification which, of course, presupposes accurate identification. Clients can now listen to the same audio recordings of their own speech that they accurately identified and quickly stop the forward movement of the tape as soon as they perceive the stuttering. Another way, when the tape recorder lacks such a button or switch, is to use two flashlights or penlights that have instant on-buttons or perhaps a noise clicker. However it is done, the purpose of these procedures is to help clients develop the necessary rapidity of identification which will serve as the foundation upon which clients rest their ability to rapidly change their speech behavior. Clients are here reinforced for the quickness of the identification to the point where their stopping of the tape recorder or signalling with a light or sounds happens *before* or close to the beginning of the stuttering. Once again, clinicians should practice this themselves until reasonably confident that they have the ability to quickly and accurately recognize their client's stuttering. Remember, try to practice the same things yourself that you ask the client to do. After sufficient practice, with a variety of stutterers, you will find that you will not have to individually prepare this aspect of therapy; however, some homework has to be done prior to your doing this with the first stutterer(s) you manage.

Clients' ability to quickly stop the tape recorder upon perceiving instances of their *own* stutterings serve as the introduction into the next phase of identification: on-line analysis. On-line analysis involves the quick and accurate identification of instances of stuttering during the actual production of speech. As previously mentioned, this is no easy task since adult stutterers must identify stutterings at the same time as they are conducting a conversation with the clinician. At this point, clients may begin to really feel and express the enormity of the task that lies in front of them. The clinician must be very sensitive to this feeling on the part of the client and discuss it with the client. The clinician must also realize that the client may find it very frustrating to have conversation interrupted by on-line identification. The client may also feel rushed, pressured, or uncomfortable when so much specific attention is being paid to speech production. The clinician must discuss these feelings and let the client know that the clinician respects them. On the other hand, clinicians must not allow such respect to paralyze them from acting in a way that is in the client's best interests no matter how painful this may be to the client in the short run.

To facilitate on-line identification, it is helpful if the clinician selects as a topic of conversation something that is familiar and of interest to the client. This on-line procedure, at least at first, should be broken up into several short periods, rather than a few long sections within one therapy session. These conversation breaks and discussions of the client's successes and failures with on-line identification enable the clinician to minimize the tension (both physiological and psychological) that build up with the therapy procedure. Better to provide the client with a few successful periods within a therapy session than to spend an entire therapy session working the client in such a way that the client is nearly driven from therapy. And make no mistake about it, clinicians, no matter how unintentionally, can drive clients away from therapy. Once again, the clinician's sensitivity regarding the client's ever-changing needs and feelings will dictate the success of this as well as other approaches. With on-line analysis in particular, where the attention to speech production is quick, pointed, and apparent, the client can easily get the feeling that all the clinician cares about is speech. The client may also get the feeling that the clinician is picking on the client. It seems in this situation that the essence of the client's reaction is that the clinician only cares about speech and not about him or her as a person. It is important to recognize this reaction as it is developing and then to discuss and possibly mitigate it.

One way we have successfully employed on-line identification with adults is by a simple contest between clients and ourself. We would begin, after conferring with clients, to specifically target certain disfluencies that clients need to identify in their own speech. Then, while we discuss with clients some topics of interest or familiarity, we try to see who is the first one to identify these specific disfluencies. Although we can signal such identity with a simple finger pointing or raising gesture, a penlight with an instant on-off button is also an effective signalling device. The objective of this contest is the speed with which the client can identify the disfluency. Obviously, clinicians can manipulate their latency of signal to maximize, at least at first, the clients' chances for identifying their own instances *before* clinicians do.

I'm beginning to stutter more

As the client becomes more and more adept at quick and accurate identification, clinician latency can be shortened to make the task more and more challenging for the client. At this point, one of several things may be noticed: (1) clients claim they are stuttering more, (2) clinicians notice clients stuttering more (possibly, because clients are avoiding less), or (3) the duration of each instance of clients' stutterings seems to be shortening. The third observation is, as previously mentioned, a positive sign that clients are improving in their objective awareness of stuttering and are already, even without direct modification procedures, beginning to change their speech production. The former two observations, however, are a bit more worrisome to both client and clinician and need some attention at this point.

We have previously discussed the client's claim that he or she is stuttering more, and we will not belabor the point at this time. Suffice it to say that clients' heightened awareness of their stuttering heightens their awareness! Stutterers believe they stutter more, we believe, because they are now becoming more objectively and accurately aware of the fact that they stutter. It is more difficult to understand why the clinician may believe that stutterers are increasing their stuttering. To be sure, the client may be stuttering more now if for no other reason than the fact that he or she talks more as the client-clinician relation develops and the client becomes more willing to enter into (less apt to avoid) discussions. On the other hand, the clinician, as well as the client, changes with therapy and becomes more adept at perceiving instances of stuttering. Further, the clinician becomes more aware, with exposure to the client, of the depth and breadth of the client's stuttering; that is, in the beginning the clinician often misses some of the client's disfluencies because the clinician must attend to a myriad of factors in the development of a reasonable evaluation and prognosis.

We find it very interesting that clinicians often report increases in their client's stuttering and express worry that they caused these increases! We doubt if they have the same worry if they notice after several sessions with a child producing articulation errors that the child is producing more such errors. Likewise, we would bet that clinicians do not have the same worry when they notice after several sessions with a child with language concerns that there is a decrease in the child's MLU or that there are more missing grammatical morphemes. What is being said here is that more or less stutterings noticed by the clinician after a period of therapy does not mean the client has gotten worse. It may simply mean that (1) the original estimates of stuttering were inaccurate; (2) that the client is talking more and in longer units; (3) or that the situations in which the speech is elicited during therapy are different from the original evaluation; or (4) any of these reasons and more in combination. Clinicians must stop flailing themselves when they notice such changes. They should attempt to make the same reactions to increased stuttering that they make to increased articulation errors, or missing grammatical morphemes, or decreased MLU, or more prevalent hoarseness, and so forth (for further discussion pertinent to this issue see Wingate 1971). Guilty parents are difficult enough to deal with, but guilty clinicians, especially when there is no reason for such guilty feelings, are even more problematic. The white, hot spotlight of on-line identification seems to exacerbate these concerns, but it is quite unclear to me how we can assist our adult client's stuttering if the client and ourselves are afraid to carefully examine, and touch, and hear those behaviors that are in error and need changing. Perhaps it is much like asking a garage mechanic to fix the engine of our car *without* examining it closely and touching and listening to it during the exam.

the bridge between identification and modification

The client's ability to temporally beat the clinician at identifying instances of stuttering is the bridge between identification and modification. With careful explanation, clients should come to understand and physically *feel* the basic things they do wrong during speech as they are doing them. I want to stress that the key here is: *as he is doing them*—not three seconds later or five words ago, but right here and now, right at the exact moment of stuttering rather than later. The physical feelings of interfering with speech and the rapidity of these behaviors must be carefully examined and accurately recognized. Once again, we stress that the problem is not within the sound or syllable but within the strategy used by the stutterer to produce those units of speech.

For some adult stutterers, simply identifying stutterings as they are being produced is sufficient to enable them to start modifying these very same instances of stuttering. That is, on-line identification of stutterings while they are being produced facilitates some adult stutterers' attempts to change stuttering. The first sign of such facilitation is a decrease in the duration of the stuttering which seems to indicate that stutterers realize that they can change their stuttering in midstream, that they can use less tension in the production of a particular sound or sound-to-sound transition. Another sign is when the stutterer in the middle of producing a stuttering stops, perhaps briefly pauses, and then initiates the same sound or syllable in a more appropriate fashion. These signs essentially mean that adult stutterers are taking an active, direct approach toward the coping with or changing of their stuttering. The stutterers give the impression that they are beginning to come to grips with their stutterings by shortening the duration and/or stopping and reinitiating in a more fluent manner. Adult stutterers give signs that they are beginning to do battle with their stuttering, rather than running and hiding or avoiding the situation. To be effective in this battle, we try to arm the adult stutterer with an objective understanding of stuttering as well as an ability to quickly and accurately confront instances of stuttering. Every time I see an adult stutterer begin this self-confrontation process, I am reminded of what I think is a Pogo quote that goes something like, "We have met the enemy and he is us." Rather than ducking and weaving, the adult stutterer has started to circumscribe the real boundaries of his or her speech problem. The client can now begin to operate from a position of understanding rather than ignorance, one of relatively clear vision rather than hazy insight.

if identification fails to develop

Some adults who stutter never seem to develop the ability to identify and subsequently modify instances of stuttering. We are not sure why this is, but several reasons may exist. First, for some, there is so much emotionality associated with the actual sight, sound, and feel of their stuttering that these individuals find it extremely difficult to actually confront occurrences of their own stuttering. Many times these clients try to keep therapy on a subjective, discussion basis (see Johnson 1946 for discussion of individuals who employ high levels of abstraction), rather than a get-down-to-specifics approach. At times, a break from therapy helps, where the clients are given some time to think about whether they are willing and able to specifically confront instances of stuttering. Secondly, other adult stutterers do not appear to have the ability to concentrate to the degree and for the length of time necessary to identify and modify instances of stuttering. Thirdly, some adult stutterers may be able to see and hear instances of stuttering but appear unable to physically *feel* these same instances. It is as if this third group of clients are physically as well as emotionally insensitive, or out of touch with their own bodily feelings. Of course, the possibility also exists that the clinician is not very effective in assisting the client identify instances of stuttering or that the clinician has not sufficiently and clearly explained the rationales for identifying instances of stuttering. We need to face the reality of the fact that some clients cannot easily, readily, or accurately perceive their own instances of stuttering and that they either need different approaches or must wait until such time that they are more receptive to our therapeutic approaches.

modification: beginning considerations

In a sense, the actual modification of stuttering is quite easy, it is just that neither we nor our clients appear to realize this fact! What is hard, on the other hand, is providing the necessary intellectual and/or emotional environment in and around the client which *continually* fosters and encourages modification of stuttering. Quick, accurate identification of stuttering is one important aspect of this environment. So is the notion that specific speaking strategies, rather than specific sounds, are the reasons for stuttering. The client must understand that stuttering involves an interference with or disruption of the smooth, easy flow from one articulatory gesture to another. Emphasis is on movement from one posture to the next, and to the next. Speech is something produced by the speaker and as such is something the speaker can modify and change. For example, a simple waltz employed by most couples on a dance floor was not so simple when they both first learned to dance. In the beginning they practiced with and without a partner the basic box, or rectangular, step until they felt reasonably comfortable with it. They practiced the specific movements of body, legs, and feet as well as placement of arms and hands. They did not practice waltzing because this would be too vague, too macrocosmic a behavior to learn. Instead, they practiced the specific movements and postures of waltzing. The end product was not as important as insuring that each subpart of the act of waltzing— this foot moves here, the arms are placed like so, and the leg or foot follows like that—was correct and properly sequenced in time. The beginning dancer knew that once he or she had accurately learned these various components, the end-product (waltzing) would be adequate and that with further time and practice, he or she could become a better and better dancer.

Well, this dancing analogy is not quite identical to changing maladaptive speaking behavior and replacing it with appropriate speaking behavior; however, neither is this analogy that far removed. That is, the adult stutterer needs to focus on the specific postures and movements and be able to initiate them or change to them when he or she so desires. If such movements and postures are produced, the end-product (speech) will be appropriate, not excellent at first but adequate and hopefully, with time and practice, better and better. Helping our adult clients focus on their speech behavior and breaking this behavior down into its constituent parts is one of our primary responsibilities in therapy. Toward these ends, Webster's (1975, 1978) work with fluency targets is a move in the right direction; however, it is assumed that future research will more clearly circumscribe those aspects of stuttered speech production in need of changing as well as those aspects of fluent speech production in need of adopting.

modification: where and what to begin changing

With adults who stutter, we first emphasize in our modification approach those aspects of speaking which are the most apparent, longest, and clearly disruptive to the forward flow of fluent speech. If we wanted, we could start with less apparent, shorter, and less physically tense speech behavior; however, most of these lesser stutterings will escape the attention of most stutterers, at least at the onset of therapy. Thus, we have found it better to start modifying the more easily recognizable stutterings because once change is effected with these stutterings, it is much more noticeable to the stutterers and their listeners. What is *easily recognizable* stuttering? This is not something that is readily explained on paper, but it is most likely a longer stuttering in association with apparent physical tension in and around the face, neck, and upper chest. Along these lines, however, we would like to point out that it is not usually necessary to *directly* remediate such apparent behavior as lack of eye contact, turning of the head, or constricting of the external throat muscles. These inappropriate behaviors are most likely a reaction to, rather than cause of, instances of stuttering. Therefore, when modifying stuttering itself (the actual disruptive speech behavior), the basis for these inappropriate reactions will diminish which means that the reactions themselves will drop out. We must remember that there are just so many hours during the therapy day and that one must pick and choose wisely in order to maximize the effectiveness and efficiency of such therapy. Thus, starting with eye contact (its obvious presence would seem to be one of the reasons it is frequently selected by beginning clinicians as a behavior to modify) is not an effective use of this time when so many other speech-related events need remedial attention, for example, inappropriate lip closure, laryngeal abductory gestures, and so forth.

Audible sound prolongations are excellent places to start modification with adult stutterers. This gamma behavior (see Table 1–1) is most likely the stutterer's reaction to sound-syllable repetition and is thus a complex behavior. Careful study will show you that a restricted number of inappropriate speaking strategies are the basic physiologic correlates of these sound prolongations. You will note the relative stability of speech physiology (that is, there is little of the rather wild oscillations of speech musculature commonly associated with sound-syllable repetitions) during the sound prolongation, but you will also notice the relatively high degree of physical tension in the speech musculature associated with the prolongation. Listening to the sound prolongation, you may hear either little or no sound (high probability but not certainty that the vocal folds are closed) or whispered, breathy, or noisy vocal quality (high probability of open vocal folds). In other cases, you may hear a glottal frylike, or popping, sound (closely approximated, but to some degree vibrating vocal folds) during the sound prolongation. You may also see that the mouth (jaw, lips, and tongue) are set for the sound being prolonged but that these structures are not moving on to the next sound (the stutterer is not making the between-sound or syllable transition). During the sound prolongation we may assume that the stutterer's rib cage and abdomen are relatively locked (fixed) or if anything, slowly deflating. All these behaviors, of course, cannot be easily explained to the client and in some cases would not be of assistance even if we were to do so. However, you should be clear of their nature and frequency. Furthermore, because the rate of speech is so fast, relative to our ability to identify and modify it, in the beginning we must help the client change inappropriate behavior during or slightly after the instance of stuttering. During and after is not a place of choice but one of necessity.

modification: after then during the instance of stuttering

Let us say, for example, that the adult stutterer holds a speech posture which results in prolonging the word-initial /s/ in the word *see*. We see the physical tension in the face and neck muscle and the closing or closed eyes; yet it is less than helpful to work on these facets of the problem, regardless of their maladaptive nature. Likewise, we hear the air rushing from the lungs, through the larynx and mouth, and yet do not tell the stutterer to "take a deep breath and start over" because he or she has run out of air. Instead, we observe the lack of speech posture movement from this prolonged sound to the next one. We witness the client's failure to make the necessary transition from the /s/ to the /i/ of the subsequent vowel. We witness clients pressing their tongue tip tightly against the alveolar ridge but do not see it moving into position for the subsequent sound. Indeed, we are not witnessing a problem with producing a sound but a problem connecting sounds—a problem with going from sound to sound, rather than a problem with a particular sound. These problems of connection are based on inappropriate strategies. In the case of sound prolongations, I believe, the strategy is one of overriding a previous inappropriate strategy used for sound repetition. Rather than continue the repetitive attempts to begin or end a speech posture without making connecting gestures to the next sound (a sound repetition), the stutterer now changes the repeating gestures and instead begins to freeze the speech posture (sound prolongation). However, the outcome is the same: The stutterer fails to move on to the next sound.

Getting back to our example of the adult stutterer prolonging the word-initial /s/, we would first try to help the stutterer change or move on to the next sound while he or she is in the middle of prolonging this sound. This would be our first attempt; however, if at first, change during the middle was not possible, then we would allow the stutterer to finish the word but immediately repeat the stuttering on this word and encourage change this time. Obviously, our procedure here is nothing particularly new (see Van Riper 1973; Starkweather 1974); however, what we do believe is slightly but importantly different is that we emphasize in lay person's terms the type of speech physiology that is being inappropriately used by the stutterer. Rather than use such terms as *blocks,* or *pull-outs,* or *bouncing,* which have a place in therapy but become too vague too quickly, we try to help the client *feel,* see, and hear the exact things he or she does that interfere with speaking. We also emphasize the common thread that runs through all these behaviors and focus attention on the client's strategies, rather than the sounds being produced.

It is not easy to help the client change speech behavior in midstream, but after a thoughtful identification program, this can be implemented without a great deal of trouble. Once adult clients appear to understand what you want them to do ("When you *feel* yourself maintaining that speech position, move on to the next speech position as quickly and smoothly as possible"), we can shorthand the procedure somewhat. Rather than saying, "change" or "move on" to the client, we can simply say, "Now" at the same moment in time. In a sense we are the clients' external monitoring device helping them tune in and turn on to the type of speech behavior in error and then change this behavior by moving on to the next sound(s). Here again, the client and clinician enter into a kind of contest to see who can first recognize the stuttering. Once so recognized, the client can change. We should caution again that this procedure requires the clinician to be very supportive and sensitive to clients and their feelings. Clients must be rewarded for successive approximations to change and the clinician's "Now" must be clear but kind, rapid but not repulsive. We do not want to harass clients the same way everybody else does. Instead, we want to objectively recognize instances of stuttering and then help clients modify (on-line) while they are stuttering. We do not expect instant success with this; we do not expect perfection, but we do expect the client to give this a try. These trys will be greatly facilitated by our support, reinforcement, and understanding for the difficulty that any human being has in changing something about themselves. It is easy to say that the modification of speech is just plain hard work.

modification: when the client fails to change

If the client fails in attempts at changing inappropriate speech behavior when you clearly but politely say, "Now," do not persevere with this procedure. *Demonstrate* for the client the actual change you are referring to; do not just *tell* the client to change. Too often we seem reluctant to actually show (through actual positioning of our own lips, tongue, jaw, and larynx) what the inappropriate speech behavior is and how we are asking the client to change this behavior. Perhaps we fear that doing so may be construed by stutterers to mean we are mocking or teasing them. However, if our feelings are right towards that client, if we have demonstrated good faith to the client in terms of our sincerity to help the client change (see Chapter Six for further discussion of clinicians' attitudes), then we have little to fear on this score. Instead, we think some of our reluctance stems more from our lack of clarity regarding *what* behavior is in need of changing and *what* behavior should be substituted. This is due, in part, to our history of concentrating on stutterings or repetitions and prolongations without looking at the actual speech physiology that makes up these speech behaviors. This concentration in turn reflects past zeitgeist (spirit of the times) in the field of stuttering which in essence implied that looking at physiological aspects of stuttering indicates the looker is seeking a physiological cause of stuttering. This zeitgeist, as we can now appreciate, has led us away from a rich source of information regarding stuttering: the actual disruptions in peripheral speech physiology which are associated with stuttering. To believe that we more precisely capture the essentials of the speech physiology associated with stuttering by avoiding the term *stuttering* and instead using terms like *sound prolongation* and *sound-syllable repetition* is to believe that we have captured the essentials of oranges, lemons, grapefruit, kumquats, and so forth by calling them *citrus fruit,* rather than mere *fruit.* (See, Andrews and Harris 1964 for further discussion of how the population of stutterers may be subdivided into various different types of stutterers.) Surely, sound prolongation is more microcosmic than stuttering, but it is still too broad, still too nonbehavioral, and still too vague to help our clients help themselves become more fluent. We must strive, as recent research suggests (Freeman 1979), to become more and more *specific* in our understanding of what our stuttering clients *do* when they interfere with speech. Such specificity will allow us to become clearer and clearer in our descriptions to these clients (particularly adult stutterers who want and need such specificity) regarding what they are doing that is labelled stuttering.

modification: when the client produces real change

We know that our clients are beginning to make significant change when we notice them effecting change in maladaptive speech production strategies *during* the actual instance of stuttering. This is a rather ethereal event that is quickly over and done with as the client moves on to the next sound, syllable, or word. The clinician must, therefore, recognize such change and *immediately* reinforce it. Such reinforcement, particularly in conversation, can be somewhat disruptive to the forward flow of communication, but it is better to interrupt than to allow to go unnoticed this very positive sign that the client is changing. The actual change may even take longer than if the client had simply "bulled" his or her way through the particular speech posture. However, the client has taken it upon himself or herself to make this change, and the clinician should definitely reward this self-initiative. Further, the client's taking slightly more time, if this is the case, demonstrates an ability to deal with time pressure, to become more independent of real and perceived reasons for "full steam ahead and damning the torpedoes." In essence, these first changes by the adult stutterer are the true beginning of the end of the problem, but this does not imply a cure in the traditional sense of the word (more on the issue of cure toward the end of this chapter).

Changes in disruptive speech posture that occur during the stuttering can then be continually reinforced in restricted utterances ("Tell me everything you know about this ballpoint pen"). Provide the client a closed set of thoughts or ideas to deal with so that he or she can concentrate on these changes in stuttering to the exclusion of conjuring up elaborate conversation. Target the change or the types of disruptive speech behavior you expect or desire the client to modify. At this point, do not ask the client to attempt to change all manner of disruptive speech behavior. Failure, like success, has a way of influencing its surroundings. We stress to the client that consistent change on longer sound prolongations is a very good first step. The client may hold too long and with too much physical tension the posture for production of the word-initial sound, but the client is making real progress if he or she can consistently demonstrate a rapid, easier movement onto the posture for the subsequent sound.

It is my belief that instances of stuttering result from inappropriate strategies, rather than difficulties with particular sound-syllables, and indeed, some clients' ability to change certain instances of stuttering (for example, reduce the length of their longer sound prolongations) generalize, and they begin to demonstrate similar change in other disfluencies. This can generalize to the point where almost overnight, it seems, the client becomes markedly more fluent. We believe that this initial burst of fluency is what some workers refer to as a *false fluency* and is not to be confused with fluency which results from a more lasting appreciation of how and why speech can be modified. It would, however, be silly to look a "gifthorse in the mouth," so to speak, and reject out of hand the initial success the client has demonstrated. At this point, in therapy, words of praise mingled in with words of caution, discussion of what is going on and why are in order. Use this success to motivate clients toward the additional work that must follow. What we do need to avoid, however, is premature dismissal from therapy and/or premature shouting of Eureka! Honesty in this situation is the best short-, medium- and long-term policy, and the client should be supported and encouraged for his or her progress to date but should not have expectations raised to unreasonable heights.

○ WITHIN-THERAPY CARRYOVER

Some clients, however, seem to make change quite easily and effectively when you are monitoring their speech but seem to do little on their own, even in your presence. Here, we are not talking about a carryover problem in the traditional sense of difficulty carryingover changes in speech from one therapy session to the next; instead we are talking about carryover problems within the therapy session itself. A client who can quickly and accurately identify and then change during a disruptive speech posture *only* when you are assisting in the monitoring and changing is a client who obviously has a problem; that is, this is a client who is not ready to transfer changed speech to the external environment. First, look to the client's understanding of the meaningfulness and rationale for your procedure. Explain again, perhaps in different terms, why you are doing what you are doing and why you think it is important. Do not be afraid to travel over old ground in this case. Secondly, look to the way you are reinforcing the client for successful approximations and achievements. Does your reward seem to mean anything to the client? Does he or she seem to understand not only when but what you are rewarding? Perhaps, your reinforcements are neutral because your relation with the client is rather neutral. Perhaps you are overly businesslike and professional in manner, and the client has trouble relating to such an approach. However, this is not a call to go completely the other way and become the client's buddy. Instead, this is just a suggestion to study the aspect of your clinical dealings with the client. Thirdly, do you make it clear what elements of the client's inappropriate strategy must be changed, or do you simply say change?

Too many times, too many clinicians fail to specifically *show*, or *demonstrate*, or *do* for the client the actual behavior they want the client to achieve. Rather, they do a lot of talking about change, and a lot of telling the client to change, or lecturing the client on change. It makes intuitive sense to this writer that a client who is quite hazy about the specifics of changing speech behavior is a client who is very unlikely to make these types of changes. The client is unlikely to put out the necessary effort to make these changes. The client is not asking for nor needing a course in the anatomy and physiology of the speech and hearing mechanism; however, the client does want and needs specific instructions on how to change, for example,

> During your sound prolongations, you hold you tongue tip tightly against the roof of your mouth in the front. You then fail to move your tongue into the position for the first position for the next sound. During this time, you're also holding open your vocal cords in your voice box. I want you to begin closing your vocal folds and moving your tongue tip into position for the next sound when you physically *feel* yourself holding them in that "stuttered" posture. Like this (and you demonstrate several times).

Obviously, even the best laid plans go awry, and some clients for unknown reasons fail to make the shift from clinician-monitored change to change on their own. These clients are problematic, but some of them respond better to approaches where they are *given* a procedure to use to change their speech. These procedures are amply covered elsewhere (for example, Van Riper 1973; Wingate 1976), but they all have a common thread running through them: The client is provided with some internally or externally generated means for minimizing stuttering. The relation of these various procedures to what we are beginning to understand regarding the speech physiology of stuttering is, at best, unclear and at worst, chiefly expedient. The client achieves fluency after a fashion, but this is not to be confused with an approach where the client is viewed as the *perpetrator* of the stuttering and as such has the means to make the change. That is, if we take, as we are in this book, the approach that clients have the means to effect change within their own speech, then it makes most sense to see what they are doing which interferes with their speech and see if they can produce more and more of an appropriate strategy for fluent speech. This is not to say that all clients can and will react positively to this approach (it is doubtful that all clients can and will react positively to any approach!), but that it is the base from which we start remediating.

○ CHANGING SPEECH IN CONVERSATION

Once the adult client begins to consistently change stuttering (shortening the duration and easily moving on to the next sound) in restricted conversations and situations with the clinician, the client can begin to effect change in more naturalistic environments. Some role playing of these situations, in advance of their occurrence, may help the client deal with and become appropriately desensitized to the actual situation. Here, once again, is where a group therapy situation which runs in parallel with individual therapy is so useful. Both you and the client get to see the extent to which the client can make the change in front of the group. Selected phone calls can also be of help where clients get to test their ability to change in the presence of time pressure. Going into stores (with the cautions mentioned in the previous chapter) are also good tests and experiences. Talking to the clinicial secretary, providing he or she has the time and is willing (and has been previously briefed on the nature and purpose of this procedure), is another good experience and test. Keep these situations brief, to the point, and allow time for discussion of the results. Do not simply do this to do this, but plan it out in advance and reinforce and or critique the client after each and every experience. If this is not a successful experience, you had better go back into the clinic and spend more time on basics. Obviously, none of it will work if the client is "sleeping" between sessions.

You can get some idea if the client is changing the frequency and duration of instances of stuttering by asking him or her, "What does your wife (father, boss, teacher, and so forth) think about your speech?" "Has anyone mentioned to you any changes in your speech?" If the client reports that associates and relatives are starting to notice positive change in his or her speaking behavior, you have a good idea that positive changes in speaking behavior are taking place outside the clinic. If you can, you might give these people a call and ask their opinion regarding your client's progress; of course, this presupposes that you have previously established some minimal working relations with them. This is not snooping into your client's personal life but honestly attempting to determine if other individuals in the client's environment are beginning to notice change. Often they may note positive change when you believe therapy is at a standstill, and this provides you with encouragement to continue the therapy. Obviously, you do not make these phone calls frequently, but they can be made at appropriate times with very positive results on future therapy plans. Likewise, if such calls indicate little change, but you are noticing considerable change in the client, this also provides you with valuable information and direction for future therapy.

○ HOMEWORK WITH ADULTS WHO STUTTER

No one likes to bring home work from the office and adults who stutter are no exception. Therefore, do not set yourself up for frustration by assigning your adult client large amounts of between-therapy work. Make these assignments short and easily accomplished in a nontherapy setting, for example, the client's bedroom in front of a dressing mirror. Make these assignments such that the client can understand how and why he or she is doing them. Be sure to monitor these assignments—write down at the end of the therapy session what the exact nature of the assignment was—so that the client realizes that you are evaluating his or her completion and relative success with these assignments. If the assignments involve speaking outside the home, for example, talking to strangers, make sure that during the week the client has an opportunity to encounter strangers! If not, switch assign-ments because neglected and impossible assignments will surely influence in-clinic therapy and most often in a negative way. At the risk of redundancy, homework assignments where the client uses the phone are one excellent means to get the client to practice identifying, monitoring, and changing speech behavior. The client's number of calls can easily be counted, the client can control the length and nature of each call fairly easily, and the exercise can be readily done at home (and in some cases, at work). The point to all such homework is practice with and habituation of behavior being discussed and dealt with in therapy. A secondary point is that such home-work assignments foster an acute awareness of speech and the need to change speech. Finally, homework assignments, especially those that are successfully completed, show clients that they indeed can change the way they speak, that they actually can do something on their own to help them-selves. There is an old saying that goes, "If you want to roll the dice, you have got to pay the price," and the price the adult stutterer has to pay to achieve more fluent speech is work outside, as well as inside, the clinic.

○ SPEECH SHOULD BE AUTOMATIC OR WHY DO I HAVE
TO THINK ABOUT IT ALL THE TIME?

About the time clients are beginning to change their inappropriate speech strategies more and more on their own, they may start to show signs of backsliding. One way or another the client may express the notion that, "Your procedure works, but only if I think about it all the time. If I don't think about it, it doesn't work." This is obviously a frustrating state of affairs for both client and clinician.

While we do not have good objective information on how long after initial change in speech an adult stutterer needs to continue consciously monitoring and changing, it does seem that this period of time is longer rather than shorter. That is, there will at least be a six-month to twelve-month period of habituation of the increasingly fluent strategy as the client generalizes this strategy to more and more speaking situations with more and more success. This period of habituation will, therefore, be a period where change in speech strategy is not automatic, where clients will have to be conscious of speech and their relative success or failure at changing and monitoring. We believe that it is wishful thinking to expect anything different, to expect quick establishment of new strategies for speaking when it has taken years to establish the other, inappropriate strategies. Misleading our clients that this will be a quick, and easy, and painless process is, in my opinion, doing them a great disservice and is more of a sin than providing ineffectual therapy. It is going to take time and effort to change maladaptive, habituated speech strategies, for example, locking the respiratory system simultaneously with opening the vocal folds together with clamping the jaw and pressing lips together, that have been used to initiate speech over many years. One does not learn to drive a car in two weeks but must spend considerable time behind the wheel in various traffic and weather conditions. For example, the process of learning to drive must first involve conscious monitoring of motor behavior until the motor behaviors necessary for shifting, steering, accelerating, and so forth are established. Even when established, these behaviors will become continually refined with further experience. Learning never stops, it just becomes less noticeable.

Besides the initial lack of automaticity with changing speech, some clients want to rush out and use their newly found fluent strategies in all situations. One can hardly blame them, but this should be restricted, at first, until the client has established these behaviors in more controlled situations, in situations where the probability for successful implementation of appropriate strategies is maximized. Once again, back to the car analogy, we tell the client that after you first learn to drive, you do not want to practice during the Indianapolis 500! Instead you drive in low-traffic, side-road situations until you get more and more of the feeling for the strategies of driving. We stress patience and try to focus on success in more restricted situations. However, I also tell clients that with time and additional experience, they will be talking in more and more difficult speaking situations. At first, however, go slow; creep before you walk.

○ WHEN TO DISMISS

In an ideal world, dismissing adult stutterers or other stutterers from therapy should be like the old response parents gave their children when the youngster asked, "Mom, how will I know when I'm in love?" The sage parent supposedly replies, "Don't worry; when it's love you'll know it." That is, when an adult stutterer is ready for dismissal from therapy, we should know it. Unfortunately this is not an ideal world, and we do not always know when to dismiss our clients from therapy. Thus, we have to take an educated guesstimation which is just that: a considered hunch based on our education, training, and clinical experience.

First, is the client giving you signs that he or she is ready for a break (either temporary or permanent)? Is he or she calling in more often than in the past with excuses for not coming to therapy? Is she more regularly arriving late and leaving early? Is he expressing doubts that he is still receiving benefits from therapy? Do other adult clients begin to question why your client continues to come in for therapy because he or she is very fluent now (or seemingly exhibiting little change)? Does therapy seem to be taking more and more of a backseat, is it becoming less and less of a priority for the client (this may suggest resistance to as well as lack of motivation for further change) even though you continually attempt to remediate the client?

Secondly, has the client demonstrated with you in therapy a quick and accurate ability to identify and change instances of disfluency? Does the frequency of stuttering hover at or below 3 percent to 5 percent? (This percentage is problematic when we are making decisions with very fluent stutterers, as we discussed before.) Does the client appear interested in helping others with similar speech problems (always a good sign I believe)? Does the clinician have to give the client minimal cues before he or she begins to change? When the client does lapse back into old speech strategies, is he or she able to quickly, easily, and without much emotionality reverse course and become more fluent? Do you find yourself, if you have group therapy, using this client as a good role model for other clients?

Thirdly, is this client, although still slowly improving, able to continue making improvements on his or her own? Do you find that this client, after a longer-than-usual break from therapy (say, three to five weeks), is able to maintain progress to date or has he or she slipped back a couple of rungs? Perhaps, if you are in real doubt about dismissal, a break from therapy might be a viable alternative. This way you can see how clients can effect change on their own away from your watchful eye and the "healing" ambience of your clinical situation. Make sure, of course, in any case, that the clients understand that the door to your clinic is always open and that you will be willing to receive their phone calls and visits.

Finally, dismissal from therapy may not mean total termination of therapy. The client may not be able to receive maximal benefit from therapy at this point for a variety of reasons, for example, too many other professional and personal obligations, problems which may be ongoing but show signs of resolution in the future, and so forth. Perhaps, at some later date, it might be better to resume therapy. However, this must be handled delicately because you do not want to engender hopes of future success when you are just plain unsure. It is better, in most cases, that you keep these thoughts to yourself but make it apparent to the client that the door is always open for further discussions and consultation. In this way, I believe, the client in the future will know many times when it is right to reenter speech and language therapy.

○ FOLLOW-UP THERAPY SESSIONS

Once clients have left therapy, their work has really just begun. In their everyday world they must now try to apply the information, insights, and new behavior which they gained in therapy. For some, this nonclinical effecting of change will go fairly smoothly, but for others it will be problematic. Hopefully, our clients have been given a sufficiently sound problem-solving orientation and will be able, although not always 100 percent successfully, to independently change and adjust according to the surroundings. You should, however, let clients know that you do not and they should not expect success every time they go to speak. Now, we realize that this instruction may sound like heresy in some circles because it appears rather pessimistic, as if the client will stutter forever and ever. Well, perhaps, but this pessimistic advice is based, in my opinion, on the reality of the situation. That is, adult stutterers have taken many years to develop their speech problem and their reactions to and emotions regarding it. This type of behavioral-emotional complex will not be changed overnight, and we believe the client should be prepared for moments, hours, and days of difficulty. We said prepared, and not excused.

You can help the client through this adjustment back to normal by scheduling follow-up therapy sessions. These should be spaced far enough apart so that you are not just duplicating the original therapy plan, only under a different guise. We have found it useful to schedule our first follow-up therapy sessions about three to six months after initial dismissal from therapy and then again in another three to six months. If the client's outside-of-clinic fluency is maintained after twelve months post-therapy then the follow-up therapy visits can be spaced even farther apart. The important part here is that the client not be set adrift, that he or she has a place of contact with a caring professional who can and will answer questions and assist the client in working through problems that arise as the client becomes a more fluent speaker. And, I might add, there are problems. For example, the client's new found fluency has the real potential for influencing relations with relatives and associates. Like a child with a new toy, adult stutterers may begin to use their new, more fluent speech any and everywhere, much to the consternation of those around them. In fact, we have had, as mentioned before, situations where the relatives were complaining that clients were now talking too much! Naturally, such problems need to be discussed between client and clinician and if possible, and where necessary, between client and concerned relatives and or associates of the client. Follow-up sessions provide a natural vehicle for discussing these issues and can be used by clients to tell themselves and others, "I'll ask my clinician what she thinks about that when I see her next month." Of course, when real pressing concerns arise, the telephone can be used and once again, the client should be told that you will welcome such calls. Better to head off little problems at the start, before they develop and enlarge into bigger ones.

○ SOME PARTING THOUGHTS

In the preceding pages we have discussed our thoughts and those of others regarding the evaluation and remediation of stutterers, with particular emphasis in this chapter on the adult who stutters. We have tried, as we said at the outset, not to provide a recipe orientation but rather a "this is what needs to be considered" approach. Obviously that which we considered was derived from our experience, training, education, and biases regarding stuttering. However, we make no apologies for the selection of our considerations because all that one can do is present that which appears most appropriate, given his or her considered opinion. Needless to say, other approaches do exist, and will be developed, and should not be slighted, but given the present space and orientation of this book, we thought it most appropriate to give a *common thread approach* rather than one fractionated among a variety of approaches.

Regardless of the specific approach, the clinician's intensity of purpose, his or her concentration with task at hand, his or her ability to attend to relevant and screen out nonrelevant detail, and his or her caring for the client will determine the outcome of therapy. Certainly we have come a long way from the days when therapy for stutterers (children, teenagers, or adults) was much more of an art form than a science or a trained skill. We have begun to enter an era where the quality and the quantity of objective data regarding the problem of stuttering has developed to a point where it must, regardless of clinical persuasion, at least be given consideration. While the art of the clinician, his or her skill in handling people, expressing concern and care for the client, and so forth, can and should never be denied, neither should basic, objective information regarding the behavior we try to remediate. Granted, not every clinician can and should become an experimentalist testing out this or that hypothesis or collecting this or that normative piece of information. However, we should all try to understand the objective information that tells us more and more about the nature of stuttering and the people who stutter, rather than merely proceed ahead with clinical formulas derived from data bases which are less than firm. Thus, I believe that the future will be a time when the art and the science of stuttering therapy can become more closely aligned. As such alignment becomes more and more of a reality, we can begin to hand down, from one generation of clinicians to another, clinical procedures which are based as much on fact as they are on tradition.

We have seen, therefore, some of the complexities, the subtleties, and vagaries of the clinical management of stuttering. As mentioned before, it is my intent with this writing to help people begin to become clear regarding their points of confusion. If we can do this, if we can begin to see areas where we are uncertain, we can begin to ask questions that may lead us to answers. On the other hand, if we are certain regarding uncertain issues, we will never ask such questions because we are so certain we understand that we never need to question. Surrounded by this imperfect world, can we realistically expect that our therapy with stutterers will be perfect, that it will contain within it no points of uncertainty? I believe we cannot harbor such expectations, but we can struggle to improve and provide the best clinical services possible. I more than welcome your joining me in the struggle, for this is the material from which we formulate purposeful and interesting lives as professionals as well as people.

Adults who stutter generally exhibit the most habituated form of stuttering and many of them have had prior therapy experience with varying degrees of success. However, adult stutterers are very often rewarding clients to work with because of their motivation to change, their desire to "finally" do something for themselves, and their more refined intellectual skills coupled with their increased maturity. With adults who stutter, the speech-language pathologist must couple modification of the client's inappropriate strategies for initiating and continuing speech production with modification of the client's attitudes, beliefs, and emotions which foster and perpetuate such strategies. Adults who stutter, like all other adults, behave in ways which influence the way they think and, conversely, they think in ways which influence the way they behave.

Therapy for adults who stutter should ideally involve (1) some form of discussion ("talk therapy") to deal with attitudes, emotions, and ideas which engender and maintain inappropriate speech production strategies, (2) objective, nonjudgment identification of those strategies used to interfere with speech production and (3) systematically assist the adult in learning how to produce different fluency enhancing strategies instead. It is our belief that the adult stutterer cannot change that which they do not know they produce; therefore, relatively quick, accurate identification of inappropriate speech production strategies must precede and continue together with effective modification of the same. Furthermore, change in the adult stutterer's speech patterns may be quite sudden and occur very shortly after the onset of therapy. However, experience indicates that patience for the rather slow manner in which changes occur in adult human behavior is a virtue that both client and clinician should develop. Much can and is being done to help adults who stutter, but the length of the time frame within which this help occurs may need to be realistically assessed *prior* to initiation of therapy.

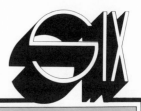

○ ORIENTATION

○ EVALUATION PRECEDES
   REMEDIATION

○ IDENTIFICATION

○ MODIFICATION

○ THE COMMON
   DENOMINATORS OF
   STUTTERERS'
   THERAPEUTICALLY INDUCED
   FLUENCY

○ THE CLINICIAN

○ FUTURE DIRECTIONS

○ SUMMARY

Conclusions

○ ORIENTATION

In the preceding chapters, we discussed the remediation of stuttering and how this remediation changes with the duration of the problem, its severity, and concomitant variables. The writer's orientation towards remediating stuttering presented during this discussion may be summarized as follows:

1. The need to recognize the importance of and develop the ability to make behavioral observations of people and their communicative and general activities.
2. The need to consider that people who stutter are people first and stutterers second.
3. The need to know what issues are typical for most stutterers but to be able to recognize important individual differences among stutterers.
4. The need to understand the speech and language characteristics of stuttering within the context of the stutterer's psychosocial concerns and makeup.

We recognize that this orientation sometimes seems rather abstract. However, this abstraction is as much due to the nature of stuttering as it is to the nature of this particular writer's orientation! It seems safe to say that in some cases abstraction is not a virtue, but of course, in other cases, neither is specificity. Clearly, it would be preferable to enumerate, quantify, and objectively specify all that we could about stuttering, but it should be recognized that this may not presently be possible or feasible, at least for certain aspects of stuttering. Thus, this writer decided not to ignore the reality of such abstract, psychosocial factors as anxiety, parental concern, guilt, and so forth. Ignoring the reality of such nonquantifiable factors would be akin to ignoring the reality of love simply because we have not as yet been able to quantify, measure, or empirically study it.

○ EVALUATION PRECEDES REMEDIATION

We have attempted to show that generating an effective therapy plan for stuttering necessitates an adequate evaluation of the stutterer, his or her stuttering speech problem, and related (non)communicative concerns. We have seen that besides stuttering (within-word disfluencies), speech-language pathologists should also recognize that various other (non)speech events need to be evaluated, for example, parental standards for child behavior as well as the child's articulation, language, voice, hearing, reading, and academic abilities. We will illustrate how difficult it is to develop such recognition by showing a classic example of the saying, "Do as I say, not as I do." In the example, it will be apparent that this writer does not himself always recognize the fact that stuttering is not the only or even principle concern of each and every stutterer he clinically serves.

Our example involves a four-and-one-half-year-old boy I was remediating for stuttering who frequently exhibited a hoarse voice quality. My ears heard, but I really did not listen to the possibility that the child's hoarseness might be a problem. Thus, I continued to focus on his stuttering. I finally woke up, to some degree, to the reality of the situation and referred this child to an otolaryngologist for determination of whether there were any physical or physiological reason(s) for such vocal symptoms. Fortunately, the physician observed no significant laryngeal pathology, but he did observe some slight superior vocal fold surface edema or reddening. This physician's observation, based on careful indirect laryngoscopy, is the type of information that one naturally expects the medical specialist to provide, rather than the speech-language pathologist. However, the physician also provided information that I, as a speech-language pathologist, would and should have known, had I not been so focused upon the child's stuttering. The physician did this by carefully questioning the mother who indicated that the *voices* I sometimes heard the child produce while waiting in the lobby (once again, I heard but did not attend) were a routine home occurrence. The child appeared to be physically tensing and straining with his vocal folds to achieve these voices (a high-pitched squeaky voice, a low-pitched froggy voice, and a loud monster voice). To compound matters, the child sometimes yelled when he produced these voices inside and outside the house. The mother was cautioned to help the child cut back on his use of these voices and unnecessary yelling.

The point of this example is that my concern for this child's stuttering clouded my judgment and kept me from asking some simple but very pertinent questions. Fortunately, in this case, the concomitant voice problem was neither serious nor apparently contributory to stuttering, but I wonder how many serious and contributory concomitant problems clinicians overlook in their realistic, but overly focused, concerns regarding a client's stuttering. Truly, an objective, thorough evaluation of our clients who stutter is something towards which we continually strive but as yet have not achieved.

○ IDENTIFICATION

If we make the reasonable assumption that the goal of stuttering therapy is to assist stutterers transfer their in-clinic fluency to the "real world," we should try to provide them with a means to insure this transfer. In our experience one such means is to have stutterers identify that which they *physically do* when they interfere with their speech production. We have previously said that it is difficult to change, on a permanent or at least a more consistent basis, that which you do not know that you do when you do it. The specificity of the identification of the interfering speech behavior would be determined by (1) the severity and nature of the stuttering behavior; (2) the client's ability to objectively and analytically assess his or her own behavior; and (3) the client's willingness to objectively grapple with what he or she does to interfere with speech.

We have previously mentioned how we help stutterers identify their interfering speech behavior by using audio and audio-visual tape recordings, mirrors, magnifying glasses, and clickers, buzzers, or flashlights (to signal to the client interfering speech behavior). We should also realize how important it is for the speech-language pathologist to have the ability to quickly, accurately, and nonemotionally point out to the stutterer the stutterer's speech behavior. This ability of the speech-language pathologist really determines, no matter what technology or equipment is used, the success of the identification procedure. The client will need to be given rationale for identification, and such rationale will have to be repeated, with more detail provided as the stutterer progresses through therapy.

Certainly, and this is an important point, identification does not and should not take the place of modification of speech production. However, identification is the beginning; it is the platform upon which we build lasting change in speech fluency. Change that passively happens to the client because of what you make the stutterer do is change that will fade with time. In clients' everyday life, when they need to change their speech, they will need to quickly and nonemotionally know how they are interfering with the forward flow of speaking behavior. It is nice to learn something, a different way of behaving, but it is even nicer, but more difficult, to know when to appropriately effect such learning. Identification provides some of this knowledge as well as a means by which the mystery and vagueness of the problem can be removed.

The objective insights gained by clients from a detailed examination of their own behavior and then rapid identification after, as well as during, its occurrence cannot be overlooked. We believe that changing the clients' speech fluency for them, without their objective awareness of what they do to interfere and what they must do to change, is a short-sighted procedure. It is a bit like expecting people to passively repeat the words, phrases, and sentences of a foreign language in the hope that they will be able to effectively use these phrases when the situation calls for their use of the foreign language. The situations and their complexities are never predictable, and neither is the learner's emotional-intellectual state when the situations arise —learners need to be able to actively generate a strategy to effect or change behavior when they realize the situation demands such action or when they are producing inappropriate behavior.

○ MODIFICATION

The 1960s brought to the field of stuttering a panoply of new terms and concepts from the area of learning theory and behavioral therapy. These terms are now relatively common to all students of stuttering, but none is more ubiquitous than the term *behavior modification*. Behavior modification, broadly defined, is a clinical procedure stemming from conditioning and learning principles used to change a client's behavior. Some have expressed the belief that behavior modification for stuttering is akin to old wine in new bottles (for example, Sheehan 1970b) whereas others appear to believe that behavior modification is one of the better, more systematic ways to remediate stuttering (for example, Ryan 1978). There is, as usual, some truth in both opinions; however, we believe that there are other issues which are just as, if not more, germane to the topic of behavior modification of stuttering.

One such topic, we believe, is this: What does an individual actually do with his or her speaking mechanism just before and during a stuttering? It would appear that in our scurry to modify stuttering, we have lost sight (if we ever saw it in the first place) of what needs to be modified! Oddly enough, after all these years of research with stuttering, we are still missing this important piece of information regarding stuttering. If we could clearly answer this question or even see the beginnings of a clear answer to this question, it would obviate much of our debate regarding which forms of remediation of stuttering are most appropriate. Indeed, the nature of the stuttering problem itself would dictate the nature of our procedures used to modify it, and this, of course, is what some people have been telling us when they advocate a particular approach to stuttering. For example, if stuttering results from or is related to a conflict in presentation of the role of the self (Sheehan 1978), then we would logically employ procedures appropriate to resolving or modifying such a conflict. Nevertheless, if we, as speech-language pathologists, hope to assist stutterers as permanently as possible to change that which they do when they stutter, it seems apparent to this writer that we need a vastly superior understanding, than that which we presently have, regarding exactly what stutterers *do* when they stutter. Telling stutterers, "You prolong the /s/ when you stutter" seems somewhat similar to telling them "You get nervous when you are anxious." A prolongation of a speech sound in time is almost by definition a stuttering and vice versa; at best, using this approach, we could describe for the client that the sound is *prolonged* and then evaluate it as a *stuttering*. However, what are we saying to ourselves regarding how the stutterer actually produced the sound prolongation? Do we talk to ourselves like we do to our clients, in this same rather vague manner of description? The answer, we are afraid, is too often *yes.*

Once again, as obvious as it seems, the nature of the speech production that is evaluated and labelled by listeners as stuttering is something that we as experts still do not clearly understand. Behavior modification might be appropriate for all stutterers if we knew exactly what aspects of the stutterers' speech production need modification! (Of course, in the strictest sense, we would have to assume that the stuttering speech behavior results from or behaves in accordance with the laws or principles of conditioning and learning.) We all can see and hear the stutterer reiterate and prolong various speech postures, but how, when, and where in the vocal tract are such reiterations or prolongations initiated and produced. At present, what too often passes for behavior modification appears to be the result of clinical expediency and or experimentation, rather than a clear knowledge of what really needs modification. This problem is compounded by some behavioral modification approaches which appear based on very rudimentary understanding of the *simple to complex* continuum of speech behavior. Many times this rudimentary understanding appears to be based more on an understanding of written, orthographic communication behavior than it does on an understanding of (dis)fluent speech articulatory, laryngeal, and respiratory behavior (see Faircloth and Faircloth 1973, pp. 77 to 78 for description of orthographic versus articulatory sounds-syllables).

A classic example of such rudimentary understanding is typified by approaches that modify speech at the isolated vowel level first and then proceed to the sentence level without apparently once considering if this progression makes sense in terms of *speech production.* We are not able to quibble with the fact that such a progression, at least some of the time, significantly assists stutterers become more fluent. However, one cannot help but wonder if such a progression is appropriate for *speaking* behavior. And it is, we must remember, *speech,* not *orthographic,* behavior that needs modification. Perhaps, if such a progression is inappropriate, it may somehow contribute to the oft-reported relapse that many stutterers experience after speech-language therapy.

Clearly, stutterers' speech needs to be modified, changed, or to coin a term, *metamorphisized.* Given this need, employing behavior modification procedures may make the most sense: These procedures are systematic, relatively quantifiable, and permit reasonably clear communication between clinicians and clients regarding therapy goals and procedure. However, to advocate behavior modification to the relative exclusion of other approaches is unwarranted, when we still are so very unclear regarding the exact etiology and manifestations of stuttering. Too often, with stuttering therapy, we have had to put the cart before the horse and provide therapy without strong justification for its use. This, of course, is understandable because we have a practical need to develop ("before all the data are in") therapy procedure despite our recognized incomplete understanding of the nature of stuttering. In this regard, stuttering is similar to cancer, where many possible causes exist but where therapies for the sake of practicality are more often based on what works, at least for a while, than they are on a clear understanding of the cause and true nature of the problem. Obviously, we must and should continue to provide such clinical services, but we should, in our writings and lectures, make it apparent that the present state of the art is less than a certain science.

Regardless of the specific approach, therapy that follows the evaluation of stuttering has two general concerns: (1) producing in-clinic change in speech behavior and related events which leads to (2) establishing outside-of-clinic change in a variety of speaking situations. Williams (1978) makes the point that the goal of our therapy with stutterers is much more importantly related to transfer of change to the outside environment than within-clinic change. Effective therapy procedures involve a continuous monitoring of the client's outside-of-clinic change and actively trying within the clinic to bring about such "real world" change. Such therapy is structured to optimize the bridge between in-clinic change and outside-of-clinic performance. Establishing this bridge is, of course, no easy task, but one that is truly the object of stuttering therapy. Assist stutterers to speak fluently in the everyday environment should they so choose, and become willing to effect the necessary behavior to engender and facilitate such speech fluency. Realistically, even if we are effective in planning for transfer of speech behavior, we should not maintain the hope that each of our clients, particularly one with a more habituated stuttering problem, will *immediately* become fluent outside the clinic. Our experience, which is consistent with Perkins' (1978) comments in this regard, is that real transfer will take longer than any of us would actually like or sometimes admit to. Speech-language pathologists dealing with stutterers would be well advised to develop patience for the length of time it takes a human being to effectively change a central or even peripheral part of themselves, especially when that part is stuttering.

We must keep in mind, however, that stuttering is not unique in terms of its relative resistance to change as a result of therapeutic intervention. In fact, human resistance to change appears to be the rule, rather than the exception, no matter if the behavior to be changed is cigarette smoking, study habits, or sexual dysfunction. For example, Zilbergeld and Evens (1980), in a critical appraisal of Masters and Johnson's (1970) sex-therapy research, state that ". . . the main problem for brief therapy is not inducing change, but maintaining it."[1] Thus, clinicians, dealing with other types of human behavior besides stuttering, in this case sexual dysfunction, are extremely concerned with the amount of relapse they observe in their clients shortly after termination of therapy. (Studies of sex-therapy relapse report, not unlike reports of stuttering-theory relapse, rates of 37 percent to 54 percent relapse after termination of therapy.)

The point of this comparison of stuttering to other human problems is to caution against suggesting to ourselves and our clients that quick cures from stuttering are readily possible. Furthermore, it appears to this writer to be unethical to encourage our clients to expect quick cures. This is not, we believe, based on current information, a pessimistic but a realistic approach to stuttering and the individual who stutters. As we mention later in this chapter, thoughts and feelings create behavior, and behavior creates thoughts and feelings. Speech-language pathologists who want to assist stutterers produce lasting change must take into consideration this circularity of influence between individuals' thinking and feeling and their behavior. When all speech-language pathologists working with stutterers, regardless of which end of the behaviorist-nonbehaviorist continuum they rest, encounter the amount of relapse in stuttering commonly observed, a need for a change in approach is obvious. We would suggest that this change reflect a movement away from the classic *t'is-t'aint* discussion between behaviorists and traditionalists towards a meld of the insights and procedures of traditional approaches and behavioral methods and principles.

○ THE COMMON DENOMINATORS OF STUTTERERS' THERAPEUTICALLY INDUCED FLUENCY

The speech behavior generally perceived as stuttering (within-word disfluencies) is readily changeable, if only temporarily. This belief is not unique to this writer but can be found expressed by other experienced clinicians, for example, Shames and Florance (1980). It is instructive, however, to briefly consider the common denominators, or threads, that run through the means by which stutterers, albeit briefly, positively change their speech fluency. A similar discussion is presented by Cooper (1978) who describes these means as *fluency initiating gestures*. Furthermore, current research in this area (for example, Brayton and Conture 1978; Adams and Ramig 1980) supports some of our hunches as well as those of fellow speech-language pathologists like Cooper (1978).

Basically, we believe that stutterers become more fluent when they minimize the sound-to-sound variability in their speech production and when they slow down the movement between, as well as within, sounds, relative

[1] B. Zilbergeld and M. Evens, "The Inadequacy of Masters and Johnson," *Psychology Today*, 14, (1980), p. 37. Reprinted by permission of B. Zilbergeld.

to normal and their own rate of utterance. Change in other variables co-occur, for example, vocal sound pressure level (Conture 1974) and fundamental frequency and articulatory contact pressure. The two variables that seem most consistently related to increments in stutterers' fluency are (1) minimized variability of speech production (homogenization) and (2) lengthening of intra- and intersegmental durations and transitions (temporal expansion). That homogenization and temporal expansion occur when stutterers become more fluent cannot be easily denied by anyone with sufficient experience with stutterers. Research clearly demonstrates that by assisting stutterers homogenizing and temporally expanding sound segment transitions and durations, they will become more fluent (see, Brayton and Conture 1978; Metz, Onufrak, and Ogburn 1979; Adams and Ramig 1980). How can we explain this situation? We cannot readily answer this rhetorical question, but some perspective can be obtained by briefly reconsidering the various philosophies of why people stutter (see, Bloodstein 1975a for more detailed coverage of these philosophies).

The *psyche philosophy* posits that stuttering is caused by nervous overflow into the peripheral speech structures and musculatures which results from an individual's psychosocial problems. Thus, there is a disruption or disturbance in the stutterer's psyche, attitudes, and beliefs, on some level, and what listener's hear and see as stuttering is nothing more than the fixations and repetitive shaking of peripheral structures and muscles manifested during other psychosocial problems. The *soma philosophy* views stuttering as the result of some inherent organic defect within the stutterer which creates speech posture reiterations and fixations but which generally differs in degree and kind from the more profound nervous system damage of a problem like cerebral palsy, which also fosters certain types of speech dysfunction. A third, perhaps *equitorial, approach* is to view the stutterer as an individual with a minimal or marginal organic defect which only becomes exacerbated or manifest when the individual speaks under certain forms of emotional, communicative, or environmental stress.

Whatever the philosophy, it does not seem terribly unreasonable to speculate that homogenizing and temporally expanding stutterers' speaking behavior should have a similar influence on their stuttering no matter how it is caused. When any aspect of our behavior breaks down, when we find it difficult to perform any complex act, or when we become concerned about our performances, we frequently go slower, minimize extent or range of movement, and draw out each movement a bit longer than normal. For example, a young child who is really trying to learn to use a spoon to pick up small pieces of food will go very slowly, be very deliberate, and exhibit a reduced range of movement. This homogenization-temporal expansion strategy seems to be a very human response to stressful situations or situations where we find it difficult (for a variety of reasons) to adequately perform a developing or newly acquired skill. We seem to simplify the behavior and perform it at a somewhat slower rate, making each aspect of the behavior as deliberate and discrete as possible. Thus, it does not seem particularly unusual that stutterers do likewise and that when they do, they become somewhat, or in some cases, completely fluent. The question remains, however, why doesn't the fluency last? To some extent it seems that the answer to this question lies in the nature of the cause of this stuttering, and this, of course, is still an unknown.

It is no surprise, therefore, that many therapy procedures which have been shown to bring about significant increments in stutterers' fluency (for example, Shames and Florance 1980; Webster 1975, 1978) employ reduction in the rate of movement between and within sounds and that variability of many aspects of speech behavior are minimized as rate is reduced. As a matter of fact, the reader is encouraged to read this sentence, one syllable per second (which temporally expands the duration of and between each syllable), and notice how difficult it is when one increases the length of each syllable's vowel to keep his or her fundamental frequency and vocal sound pressure level from becoming monotonous. Thus, for example, during rhythmic stimulation, the stutterer's variability in vocal pitch or level is minimized along with a time expansion between each adjacent syllable (Conture and Metz 1974) and of each syllable's vowel duration (Brayton and Conture 1978).

These aspects of speech production events are just now becoming more clearly understood through empirical research, but speech-language pathologists working with stutterers have intuitively known of their influence on stutterers for years. We must not, therefore, be too eager to claim novelty for such procedures and yet, on the other hand, we should not be too eager to totally cast these procedures aside, simply because they have been kicking around the back drawers of our clinical desks for years. They deserve, at least, continued, careful, empirical study and systematic clinical investigation. What we need as a discipline is more expressed commonality in approach rather than the oft-made remark that all therapies are alike, regardless of theories. If they are so much alike, we should make explicit to each other, our students, and fellow professionals how they are similar, instead of giving the appearance of vast differences in approach. One very meaningful attempt at displaying commonalities among various stuttering theorists and/or therapies is presented in an edited book by Gregory (1978). In this book, Gregory and his contributing authors discuss their various approaches to stuttering, and by their so doing the reader gains the knowledge that these clinicians do share certain common ideas despite their more well-known differences of opinion. Another, even more recent attempt (Guitar and Peters 1980) at comparing and melding behavioral and traditional approaches to stuttering suggests that others also feel some need to explore the commonalities of stuttering therapy.

While differences may be healthy and lead to constant exploration, they may also give the lay public the impression that no one really knows what is going on with stuttering. This latter public impression is, however, clearly not the case. As alluded to in the first chapter, much has been discovered in the area of stuttering, and we need to make this fact apparent, in addition to explicating the degree of similarities among our various approaches. Charlatans would appear to have less chance of dealing with stutterers, for the most part, if we who conscientiously deliver clinical services to stutterers would put more of a concerted effort into explaining how much consistency there really is among approaches to stuttering used by speech-language pathologists who specialize in this disorder. The common thread among our therapies must be there because too many seemingly different therapeutic approaches appear to have a similar ameliorative influence on stutterers' speech. If nothing else, keeping this common thread notion in mind when we evaluate and remediate stutterers should help us, as individual speech-language pathologists, clarify the problem of stuttering for ourselves. Of course, clarification of a problem is not a solution of the same, but at least it is a start.

○ THE CLINICIAN

Besides our actual approach to stuttering therapy, we must also be concerned with speech-language pathologists themselves and their knowledge, motivation, and personality for stuttering therapy. Van Riper (1975) described three personal characteristics which successful clinicians appear to possess: accurate empathy, nonpossessive warmth, and genuineness (see Appendix C for more general discussion of clinician concerns and characteristics). Briefly, empathy relates to our ability to understand or imagine how other individuals feel about themselves and things that surround them. It is the ability to "walk a mile in my shoes" that successful clinicians make so apparent. The second characteristic, warmth, is something we all feel, to greater or lesser degrees, in our daily interactions with people, and it is another feature that successful clinicians seem to exude and establish in their clinical relations. Warmth relates to the ability to imply or make explicit our desire to help our clients, to make them know we care and that we think they are O.K. (perhaps, best done when we, ourselves, can say, "I'm O.K.—You're O.K." [Harris 1967]). The third characteristic, genuineness, relates to the clinicians' openness, the ability to expose their unique human traits, and be, in essence, themselves. It is difficult to like your clients when you demonstrate in one way or another that you do not like yourself. Your clients do not expect a superman or superwoman, but they do expect you to be honest and straightforward with them regarding your assets and liabilities.

Of the three personal characteristics of a successful stuttering therapist, the one that seems the biggest challenge for normally fluent speech-language pathologists to obtain is that of empathy. Here I refer to problem-specific empathy: what it feels like to actually stutter and to be a stutterer. The old classroom practice of having undergraduates go out and stutter openly for a day or in front of ten different strangers was a small step in the direction of developing this problem-specific empathy. Surely, we can, as normally fluent speakers, empathize with people who have various problems that we do not have ourselves, but to get the real feeling of what it is like to be unable to move forward when speaking is something that is best appreciated by doing. This is by no means saying that stutterers are the only ones who can do stuttering therapy (any more than it says that heart attack victims make the best cardio-vascular surgeons). However, we are saying that normally fluent speakers must work diligently to grasp some of the feelings that stutterers have when they stutter. I, therefore, frequently ask the client who stutters: "Tell me what it feels like to stutter? Do you feel terror? embarrassment? fear? pain? hurt? frustration? a numb sensation? Is it like almost having a close accident in your car? Do you want to run out of the room? and so forth." In this way, over the years, I have gained a measure of appreciation for the feelings of individuals when they stutter. I say *measure* because truly no one can totally understand what it feels like to be someone else. We can come close, and get a pretty decent idea, but never fully know.

One way we have found that seems to closely describe the feelings of stuttering is to analogize it to the momentary panic, terror, and fear people encounter when they pull back from a ledge or high place from which they almost fell. During the physical maneuver back from the ledge, people attend to emotional elements and have little awareness of what they did that got them safely back from the edge. This *mental whiteout,* as I call it, is the worst time for stutterers to objectively concentrate on what they are doing that interferes with speech, but this is the very time they need to objectively concentrate. We try such analogies out on our clients who, we believe, may be experiencing them and see what they say.

We admit to clients our inability to totally understand everything about the problem of stuttering (an example of genuineness) but try to explain that we really want to know about the clients' feelings so we can understand the problem and help the clients help themselves (an example of warmth). It goes without saying, as Van Riper (1975) nicely points out, that the personal characteristics of speech-language pathologist who works with stutterers must be built upon a solid foundation of knowledge about stuttering and then refined through a series of experiences with stutterers. Perhaps, describing the clinician's personal characteristics is just another way of talking about the *art* of stuttering therapy. Likewise, describing the clinician's knowledge of and experience with stuttering is simply another means of discussing the *science* of stuttering therapy. When the art and the science of stuttering therapy are viewed from this perspective, it is a bit easier to see

that each is necessary, but only taken together are they sufficient for successful remediation of stuttering.

○ FUTURE DIRECTIONS

The team that loses the championship game is always quoted as
saying, "... wait until next year." Indeed, the future is generally looked
upon with hope that things will work out for the better. We, too, as speech-
language pathologists who work with stutterers, are also anticipating that
new approaches and information, "just around the bend," will improve our
clinical acumen and approach. Can we at this point, however, try to guess
what these new ideas and procedures might consist of? I think so.

First, we think that technology is advancing so rapidly (for example, see
Kiritani 1977) that information regarding speech physiology, information
which is still quite difficult to obtain and laborious to analyze and process,
will become increasingly more available. As these technologies and the
information they provide move from the basic to the applied research laboratories, our general understanding of what stutterers actually do when they
stutter will significantly increase. The current mysteries of laryngeal behavior during stuttering and the complex interactions among respiratory, laryngeal, and supraglottal articulation will be solved (see Dalton and Hardcastle
1977 for description of these interactions during fluency). With the increase
in information, more and more the question will be raised: What does this
mean in terms of therapy?

Secondly, the technology will then move from the applied laboratories to
the clinical setting where practicing speech-language pathologists will actually gather objective data on each individual client. This data will be compared to existing information regarding the speech physiology of stutterers,
and the clinician will indicate which types of exhibited disruptions of speech
physiology are associated with clinical failures and successes. Some will also
take this technology and directly apply it in remediation through means of
biofeedback and similar procedures.

Thirdly, with advances in our understanding of how stutterers actually
stutter, more and more applied researchers-clinicians will systematically
investigate the issue of transfer. Parallels will be drawn between stuttering
therapy and other therapies used to remediate human disorders, for example, sexual dysfunction, where it will become increasingly apparent that
changing of behavior is much less difficult than maintaining it. This common
difficulty, which many different therapies share, will become an increasingly
obvious concern and one to which much attention and thought will be
applied.

Fourth, the traditional therapies and the behavioral therapies will meet
in the middle. Recognizing that thought and feelings give rise to behavior

and that behavior itself can influence thought and feelings, the insightful, perhaps abstract, approach of the traditionalists will be blended with the more empirical, perhaps more specific, approach of the behaviorists. This meld will benefit from two divergent events: (1) the increasing amount of information generated from the study of disordered speech physiology and (2) the growing trend in some physical sciences, for example, biology and physics, toward more humanistic approaches to science. While the pendulum of thought in the field of stuttering will never completely stop in the middle, it is believed that the extent of its swing from one side to another will never again be quite as great as it has been in the past. Dealing with this midground will mean that students, in both their academic and clinical training, will need to be exposed to behavioral as well as humanistic studies, principles, and practices. It will also mean that they will, at least, need to be knowledgeable enough of human speech physiology to be able to read in the literature and apply such information to the evaluation and remediation of stuttering.

Fifth, and finally, individuals claiming clinical and theoretical monopolies on the truth regarding stuttering will become rarer and rarer. As the true complexities, nuances, and subtleties of stuttering become increasingly apparent to larger, more sophisticated groups of clinical-research professionals, there will be less chance that any one individual can (or will try to) claim a clinical or theoretical monopoly on the truth regarding stuttering. The facts of the matter will simply weigh so heavily against such an individual, so many professionals will recognize the untenable nature of such a monopoly, that few will dare claim one and those who do will receive scant attention. This widespread recognition of stuttering's complexities and nuances which will counter the inappropriate approaches of a few will mark the true advancement of stuttering from an interesting object to be kicked around among different disciplines into a recognized discipline with its own standards, approaches, and body of knowledge, based on objective clinical and laboratory endeavor.

Harbingers for the future of remediation of stuttering are bright. We have become increasingly more sophisticated in our basic knowledge of stuttering and our evaluation of claims of therapeutic success (for example, Runyan and Adams 1978; Metz, Onufrak, and Ogburn 1979). Such sophistication can only lead to increasingly more appropriate approaches to remediating stuttering and to research projects which will bring us closer and closer to understanding the truth about stuttering. It will be recalled from the front of this book, that readers of these pages were offered *No* guarantees, recipes, or total solutions for curing stuttering and to this writer's knowledge, none were given. Guarantees, cures, and total solutions for complex human problems like stuttering are ideals to which one might like to aspire; however, one must also recognize that such ideals are not compatible with the present state of the human condition. Recognizing the imperfections of this condition, while certainly no panacea, at least provides us with a realistic backdrop against which we can make our clinical evaluation and remediation of stuttering. We are confident that in the future, speech-language pathologists will more clearly understand the human condition that everybody, including stutterers, shares, such that in their daily dealings with stutterers, they will realize, as Niebuhr (1934) suggested, "... what cannot be changed ... what should be changed, and wisdom to distinguish the one from the other."[2]

This book has examined the nature of stuttering and how it may be evaluated and remediated according to the nature of its manifestation and the chronlogical/mental age of the client. The approach taken throughout these pages has been a behavioral, problem-solving orientation; a "this is what needs to be considered" rather than a "cookbook" or "recipe" approach. The individual who stutters was viewed as an individual first and a stutterer second; viewed within the totality of his or her existence rather than solely within the component given over to speech fluency.

Therapy approaches that seem to work, at least temporarily, seem to have common threads (besides that unknown blend of science and art employed by all successful clinicians): (1) temporal lengthening of intra-and intersegmental durations and transitions (temporal expansion) and (2) minimized variability of speech production (homogenization). The clinician who has a suitable personal approach (one who exhibits empathy for the feelings of others) and who possesses an adequate technical understanding of stuttering can effectively employ one or both of the above "common threads" (as well as other procedures) and achieve reasonable results. Obviously, however, for a speech-language pathologist to arrive at a point where "reasonable results" with most stutterers are commonplace takes some clinical experience and perseverance in addition to appropriate technical/professional knowledge and interpersonal skills. Furthermore, the clinician who works with stutterers must be a keen observer of human behavior and attitudes and be able to change procedure according to the needs of the clinical situation. Indeed, recognizing what needs to be changed is no more important than recognizing what can be changed.

[2]J. Bingham, *Courage to Change: An Introduction to the Life and Thought of Reinhold Niebuhr* (Boston: Little, Brown, 1961), p. iii.

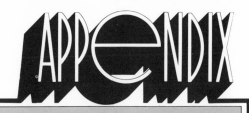

○ A QUESTIONS TO BE ASKED DURING INTERVIEW OF THE PARENT(S) OF A DISFLUENT CHILD

○ B THE ONSET OF STUTTERING: A CASE STUDY

    introduction

    procedure

    the interview

    discussion

○ C NOTE TO A BEGINNING SPEECH-LANGUAGE PATHOLOGIST

    clinicians as people

    a clinician's need to be self-analytical

    a personality "suitable" for becoming a clinician

    the development of a clinician: from classroom to clinic

    how much training you have had

    "my child's been with *you* for three months and I don't see any change"

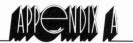

○ QUESTIONS TO BE USED DURING INTERVIEW
OF THE PARENT(S) OF A DISFLUENT CHILD
(may be adopted to use with older children and adults)

What can we do to help you? or Tell us (me) about why you are here today? or Tell us (me) about the (your child's) problem? or What seems to be the matter or the problem?

Tell us a little about his or her general development (from birth to present). (Do not strive for detail at this point.)

How does this compare with the development of his or her sister(s) and brother(s)?

Other children his age that you may know? Are you satisfied with his or her development?

Are there any speech, hearing, or language problems in other family members (mother's *and* father's side) or relatives? (If so) did they receive speech therapy or other professional assistance (help)?

When did he or she begin to babble (you may need to define the term babbling)?

Begin to imitate (non)speech sounds?

Begin to say first words?

Begin to say first phrases? (for example, "milk all gone")

Does he or she have any articulation or language problems?

How is he or she performing in school? (Be sure to know if child is in school before asking this question.)

Which subjects does he or she like the best?

How does he or she do in these subjects?

Which subjects does he or she like the least?

How does he or she do in these subjects?

What are his or her interests or hobbies?

Who are his or her playmates? Ages? (Are they younger or older?)

(At this time you may present selected items of the Vineland Social Maturity Scale or else intersperse them during the interview.)

Is there anything (other than speaking) that particularly concerns you about your child?

Describe what you see to be your child's speaking problem(s) at this time.

154

When did this start?

Who noticed the problem first? Under what circumstances?

Were you worried or concerned about it at the beginning?

What did you do about it?

Did you bring this problem to his or her attention?

What did you call it?

When did *you* begin to use the word stuttering?

If not you, who did?

Did you or do you ever notice the same behavior in your other children at any time?

Children of relatives, neighbors, and so on?

Did your child have any trouble saying words? Sounds? Letters? Does he or she now? (Articulation, and so on?)

Describe your child's speech (stuttering) behavior as it was prior to now.

Is it the same now?

Has it changed? (that is, duration, type, frequency—cyclical—stabilized)

It may be necessary to provide examples, for example, sound repetition, sound prolongation; word, part-word or phrase repetition—Clinician should know how to produce these various disfluency types.

Any body movements? Before? Now? (Other concomitant behaviors?)

Eye contact? (Has this changed since beginning of problem?)

Facial grimaces?

What aspect of the problem concerns you the most?

What was or is different that the child had or has never done before?

Since the onset of this speech problem has your child done this every time he or she has spoken? Is he or she ever fluent?

Is he or she ever more disfluent—

Anxiety———— in certain situations?
                on any particular words? sounds? letters?
Situational   with certain listeners? for example, authority figures
Hierarchy——— strangers, friends, mother, father, and so on

Does he or she avoid any situations so to avoid speaking?

What is your theory(ies) of why stuttering (this speech problem) developed?

Do you expect it to change?

How?

If it were to change—do you think there would be any other changes in various aspects of his or her behavior?

Would the child be different (for example, interaction) if he or she did not stutter?

What have you been told previously about your child's stuttering? Other problems? (Advice from relatives, teachers, friends, doctor, speech pathologist, and so on.)

Has your child had any speech therapy? Other counselling? (Has anyone else in your family had any kind of counselling, for example, psychological? academic?)

If you could wish for three things for your child (the sky is the limit), what would you wish for?

What have you done to help your child stop stuttering?

Does or did it help?

Who recommended this?

Why do you do this?

Do you think that your child reacts to his or her speech behavior? (Does he or she get embarrassed or show concern?)

Is he or she aware? How do you know?

How does he or she react to your recommendations, prompting, help?

Does your child try to improve his or her speech?

Results?

How do you react to your child's stuttering? (For instance, looking away, speaking for him or her, interrupting, punishing?)

What about children, relatives, friends, strangers, and so on?

Is someone or others more critical of his or her speech?

How do you react when your child is speaking in front of others?

Do other children ever tease your child about his or her speaking?

How does he or she react to this teasing? How do you react? (Does this teasing hurt you?)

What kinds of things do you do as a family? What does your child enjoy most? The least?

* Do you talk with your child very much? (read, play, and so on.) Your spouse?

How does the child get along with sister(s) and brother(s)? Any hostilities, or jealousies, or rivalries?

How do you (or your spouse) handle these?

Does your child play well alone?

With others?

Does he or she have many friends? Do they visit him or her at home? Does he or she visit them?

Does the child require much attention? More than normal? Needs more from mother or father?

How does he or she adjust to a new environment, situation? Sensitive to changes in environment? routine? discipline?

How does the child react to discipline? How do you, in general, discipline? (Stress need for information and that you are not going to discipline them for their discipline procedures!)

*This is an important question—dwell on it if there are hints of inadequate parent-child or parent-parent communication.

Does he or she do what you ask? Complete chores, and so on?

Does he or she do anything that particularly annoys you or anyone else? Why does it annoy you? How have you attempted to resolve this problem?

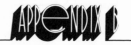

○ ONSET OF STUTTERING: A CASE STUDY

introduction

There are many factors that influence the detail and dependability of information gathered regarding the nature of events surrounding the onset of stuttering. One important factor is the interval of time from the onset of stuttering to the first interview between the parents of a stuttering child and a speech clinician. The speech therapist, in most cases, has to rely on the memory of parents about their reactions to and events concomitant with the beginnings of the stuttering problem. Any factor(s) that might dull parental memories, such as the length of time between the onset of stuttering and the parents' recollections about this, would, of course, interfere with the clearest possible understanding of the onset and development of stuttering.

The importance of the time interval between the onset of stuttering and the first interview was stressed by Johnson and others (1959). In Johnson and others' studies on the onset of stuttering, it seems that attempts were made to study "stuttering cases . . . in whom stuttering was of recent origin."[1] These workers apparently felt that the shorter the time period between onset and interview, the more detailed and dependable would be the information concerning the onset of stuttering. Even so, the median interval between date of onset of stuttering and date of initial interview (in the earliest study) was five months and eighteen days. In a later study, the median interval was seventeen to seventeen and a half months (the exact median interval being dependent upon whether one uses the mother's or the father's report of the date of onset). The shortest interval for the first study was four days; for the later study, the shortest interval was less than one month. Therefore, even though Johnson and his coworkers interviewed a few cases within a short interval after onset, that is, one month or less, the bulk of the cases was seen several months to a year after onset of stuttering. The fact that parents, in general, wait awhile before bringing their stuttering child to a speech therapist may say something in and of itself about the nature of the onset and development of stuttering. Whatever the case, our

[1]W. Johnson and others, *The Onset of Stuttering* (Minneapolis, Minn.: University of Minnesota Press, 1959), p. 15. Reprinted by permission.

understanding of the onset of stuttering would be enhanced if we could interview parents and their children as soon as possible after the reported beginnings of stuttering.

In general, we are seeking to provide further information about the nature of the onset of stuttering. Specifically, we present a detailed account of a mother's and father's description of their son's incipient stuttering problem. This account appears uniquely capable of at least partially achieving the previously stated purpose for two main reasons: (1) the time interval between the reported onset and the initial interview was only eight days, and (2) the parents had discussed between themselves and written down the events surrounding the beginnings of their son's speech problem.

procedure

The parents, Mr. and Mrs. F. (the father was 52 years of age and the mother was 37), were interviewed both separately and together. Their son, age three years, eight months (he will be called Sammy here) was separated from his parents during the majority of this interview. It was not possible to do an extensive hearing evaluation or intelligence testing because of limits on the parents' time. Therefore, it was felt that the available time would be most profitably spent in questioning the parents (especially the mother, who had apparently first diagnosed her son's speech as being stuttered) about the onset of the stuttering problem and about their son's speech and language development in general. Informal evaluation of the child's articulatory, phonatory, and language usage (formal testing of these areas was impractical since the child was uncooperative and also cried during much of the time he was separated from his mother) did not suggest the presence of any problem(s). One whole-word repetition was noticed, but this was not considered unusual for a child of three years, eight months. In short, Sammy appeared to be well within normal limits for a child his age in the areas of motor, intellectual, and speech-language development (once again, it should be noted that such statements were made on the basis of informal evaluation and not from formal testing). At the end of the interview, the parents were counselled regarding 1) the findings of the diagnostic and 2) their future management of their son's speech problem.

the interview

The mother, who did the majority of the talking for both parents, was asked to describe, from the beginning, the events surrounding the onset of the stuttering problem. Mrs. F. said that she had first noticed something wrong with Sammy's speech on the night of Monday, 1/31/72 (the date of the first interview was Tuesday, 2/8/72). At that time the family was watching the television program *Laugh-in,* when a person on the program began mocking a stuttering person. Shortly thereafter, the mother said she noticed Sammy stuttering in apparent imitation* of the television character. The mother reported that neither she nor her husband said anything to the child about his speech behavior, but Mrs. F. said that she did look very shocked, an expression which she was sure her son had noticed. The mother then recalled that she had remarked to her husband, in the presence of their son, "Did you hear that?" in reference to Sammy's speech behavior. The father then replied to the mother, still in Sammy's presence, that the boy had done the same thing just a minute ago. However, both parents reported that neither of them had, at that time, mentioned anything directly to their son about his speech behavior. Neither parent could say for sure whether, when Sammy's stuttering was first noticed, he was using force or more effort than usual to produce speech. The mother did report that for the next two days she noticed the child producing several disfluencies, but she still did not mention these disfluencies to her son. During these next two days, Tuesday, 2/1, and Wednesday, 2/2, Mrs. F. said that she noticed the child several times repeating the word *mother* or prolonging the initial /m/ of the word *mother.* On the third day, Thursday, 2/3, the mother reported that she got frustrated with her son's speech. She reported that on this day, if her son would begin to repeat a syllable or word, she would yell at him to "shut up and start over again." Mrs. F. also reported that on that day she told Sammy to "stop talking that way" when she noticed him repeating a sound or a word. (The mother's frustration with her son's speech behavior is probably what led her to call the writer on the phone that day, Thursday, 2/3. In our telephone conversation, she expressed her concern about her son's speech and referred to his problem alternately as stuttering or double talk.) All of these scoldings and reprimands, the mother reported, resulted in Sammy's crying. (However, the mother commented that he would start to cry whenever she would even "look cross-eyed at him.")

Both parents described their son's speech problem as being cyclical in nature, that is, some days he stuttered more than other days. The mother felt that most of her son's trouble developed at the beginning of a sentence he was formulating about something that was new or unclear to him. At these times, Mrs. F. said that he would repeat the first syllable of the first word or two of the sentence until he "got his train of thought." When questioned about the cyclical nature of their son's stuttering, the parents gave the following examples: Saturday, 2/5, the mother was home alone with the child and only one stuttering was noticed; however, on Sunday, 2/6, when the father was home alone with the child, Mr. F. reported that Sammy stuttered all day.

*Even after intensive questioning, neither mother nor father could clearly describe the nature of this imitation; the only thing the mother could say was that she was so shocked at Sammy's stuttering that she could not remember the exact nature of the stuttering.

When the parents were asked for their opinion as to why their son had a speech problem, the mother responded that Sammy stuttered primarily because he imitated the television performer. However, Mrs. F. stated that the imitation might have "brought to the surface some quirk or defect in his brain" that maintained the stuttering response well after the initial imitative response. The mother felt that some *quirk or defect* would have to be present to explain why her son had remained disfluent as long as he had.

The mother described Sammy as being in need of constant attention from her (she called him her "constant shadow"). She also felt that Sammy was very aggressive since he was constantly hitting his older siblings or pestering the cat. The mother, reportedly, attempted to deal with her son's misconduct by yelling or screaming at him. (Mrs. F. stated that she never hit any of her children. Sammy was the last of her four children, and only the three younger children still lived with the parents.) Sammy reacted to this yelling, according to the mother, by crying, getting upset, or by telling his mother, "Don't yell at me." Both parents described their son's motor, social (for example, toilet training), and speech development as being essentially normal.

In general, the father's responses to most questions about his son's development suggested that he was not overly concerned with any facet of Sammy's maturational progress and, in fact, seemed to believe that his son was essentially normal for his age. However, the mother felt that Sammy was somewhat slow in his overall development, and she also felt that he could behave better. On the other hand, Mrs. F. commented that she was unable to see how her son's speech could be defective when the rest of him was "perfect." In fact, the mother indicated considerable concern over the fact that Sammy might be less than perfect in something, since everyone in his family always "tried to be perfect in everything they did."

When questioned with regard to whether they had any relatives with speech problems, the father said that his 30-year-old son (by another marriage) began to stutter when he was fourteen years old. Mrs. F. said that she thought that her husband's son, even as an adult, was "hesitant when he talks." The mother went on to report that her sister's daughter had a speech problem when she was young, that is, her speech was very unclear and difficult to understand. Neither parent reported any major trauma or accident, either psychological or physical, that Sammy had ever been involved in.

discussion

From the information gathered during this interview, it can be stated that nothing seemed to be grossly wrong with Sammy, either psychologically or physiologically. Further, there were no apparent speech or language problems; that is, the child appeared to be articulating speech and receiving and expressing linguistic messages adequately for a child of his age. What, then, was the problem? This author believes that it was just such normalcy of development that led the parents to react to their son's speech. That is, as Johnson (1961) points out, ". . . parents are most likely to decide their children are stuttering when they are hesitating and repeating for no reason that the parents can detect."[2] This hypothesis seems to have even more merit when it is remembered that the mother did not become really concerned with her son's speech until the third day after the initial imitative response. At first, both parents were relatively tolerant of the child's speech problem because they felt he was simply imitating the television performer, but when the child persisted into the third and fourth days, the parents (the mother primarily) both started to worry over and react to the child's speech behavior. (Further support for this idea comes from the fact that the mother reported that she at first described the child's speech behavior as double talk and that it was not until the third day that she realized he was stuttering!)

Of course, the parental admonitions to "shut up and start over again" fit into the Johnsonian *diagnosogenic model* (Johnson, and others 1967) in that now the parents were reacting to their own diagnostic label of stuttering. And, of course, as the model would predict, Sammy might

> . . . learn to doubt that he can talk smoothly enough to please the people he talks to, mainly his parents. . . . What this amounts to is that he learns to be afraid that 'he will stutter' and that if he does he, along with "the stuttering," will be disapproved.[3]

However, in the present situation, the child hopefully will never get to the point where he has learned to react to his parents' reactions to his speech by attempting to avoid stuttering. This may be the case since the parents were given the following:

1. information regarding the normal development of speech and language, es-pecially the period during which children are normally disfluent;
2. advice to listen to the *content* of the child's expressions instead of to *how* the child expresses himself;
3. advice to reduce the psychological tension and stress placed on the child when he does not do exactly what is expected of him;
4. advice to allow the child to talk as much as possible without any attempt to change the content or manner of his verbalizations.

Further, in attempts to clarify the proceeding points, the parents were given a copy of W. Johnson's (1949) "An Open Letter to the Mother of a

[2]W. Johnson, *Stuttering and What You Can Do About It* (Minneapolis, Minn.: University of Minnesota Press, 1961), p. 126. Reprinted by permission.
[3]Ibid., p. 68.

Stuttering Child." (Currently we might also use Ainsworth's [1977] or Cooper's [1979] pamphlets.) It was felt that the parents' level of understanding was such that, following the informal counselling they received from this writer, they would be able to derive benefit from Johnson's "Letter." The parents were instructed to check back with the author in six months, no matter what the status of their son's speech and language development.

In conclusion, even within the limits of the interview procedure, it would appear that the short time interval between the date of onset of stuttering and the first interview in this case probably enhanced the detail and dependability of the information derived concerning the onset and development of Sammy's stuttering. Of course, such factors as low intelligence or hearing loss cannot be ruled out as contributing factors, but as already mentioned, the probability that such factors are contributory appears to be slight. Further, the information procedure would appear to strongly support the diagnosogenic model of the onset of stuttering. This does not imply that some other model might not adequately explain the findings with regard to the child's onset of stuttering. However, it does suggest the viability of the hypothesis that stuttering finds its beginnings or onset in parental reactions to the child's normal developmental disfluencies.

It must be emphasized that before we are ever to get a clearer understanding of the origins of the stuttering problem, we must procure more and more cases like Sammy's in which effects of time have not had a chance to erase the necessary details. For as long as we are to deal with human memory and human biases, as it appears we must when we attempt to understand the onset of stuttering through interview techniques, we must attempt to eliminate all factors that tend to cloud and distort human recollections about past events and perceptions.

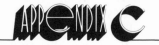

○ NOTE TO A BEGINNING SPEECH-LANGUAGE PATHOLOGIST

clinicians as people

Before we became speech and language clinicians, we were people, and we will be people after we stop being clinicians. We need to know as much about ourselves as people as we do about communicative disorders if we really want to become effective clinicians. This is not a plea for encounter sessions, T-groups, psychoanalysis, and the like (even though some of us, from time to time, may need and seek such experiences), but it is a plea for the need to consider ourselves as people, people with frailities, people with strengths, people who are constantly learning how to facilitate learning in other people and hopefully, ourselves.

Many of the problems that parents bring to us are problems we still wrestle with within ourselves. Many of our young clients' concerns we had as children ourselves or are concerns we have with our own youngsters. We should not feel helpless knowing these things. Instead, we may feel some relief that our clients share in the same human condition that we are experiencing.

Starting from a base where we recognize our humanness and all that it entails, we have a lot less farther to fall when we come up against the difficulties of changing certain aspects of the human condition. Let us then consider some aspects about ourselves that will play a factor in our dealings with clients with communicative disorders.

a clinician's need to be self-analytical

Somewhere between total oblivion to our mistakes and complete paralysis if a mistake is made is the area that clinicians should strive for. Happy-go-lucky clinicians who bumble through diagnosis and management are constantly amazed that their performances are not always the best. Conversely, clinicians who are paralyzed with fear that they will make a mistake are constantly amazed that they ever do anything right.

The ability to be appropriately self-analytical is a skill that is not easily acquired, but it is a skill well worth the acquisition. Clinicians who are continually growing, in the professional sense are the clinicians who are capable of turning the errors they produce back into the system. Many clinicians resist the development of self-appraisal skills for a variety of reasons, none the least of which is the real threat to self that such personal scrutiny represents. Such clinicians are often confused between their *self* (personality) and their *behavior.* These clinicians can advise Mrs. Jones to tell Tommy, "I do not like having orange peels thrown on the rug" instead of the usual, "Tommy, why are you such a bad boy." However, these same clinicians cannot apply this logic to their own self-analysis.

Knowing when you are going in the right or wrong direction is fundamental to your continued improvement as a clinician. Surely, other professionals and personnel will tell you how you are doing and if they like or dislike your work, but if you are *totally* dependent upon them for your feedback and monitoring of performance it is going to be a long, long time before you start to see substantial improvement in your performance. You have to really work at developing an objective appraisal system for your *own* performance. It will not come overnight. You will have to develop sensitivity for other peoples' *unspoken* feelings, ideas, and so forth and change your performance accordingly. You will have to be a better reader of clinical situations and adapt yourself appropriately.

Obviously, self-analysis will, from time to time, indicate to you that you are in error. Knowing you are in error will require you to modify your performance. Your ability to modify and entertain the notion that you are in error will take maturity and compromise on your part. The temptation to negate your errors and assign the blame to your client, the parents, your supervisor, your professors, the system, and so forth will be great. However, such passing of the buck will not allow you to fully develop to the greatest extent possible. You will have to shoulder the responsibility for your errors and performance and attempt to appropriately modify them.

The monitoring of your clinical performance requires diligence but not necessarily paranoid caution. You can be relatively flexible in clinical situations as long as you realize that you are capable of changing your inappropriate clinical procedures. Your ability to monitor and change is as much an assumption for you as for your client—if you cannot monitor and modify your own behavior, how do you expect your client to do so?

a personality "suitable" for becoming a clinician

Interpersonal relations are obviously of importance to the speech-language pathologist. The personality of the clinician does enter into the clinical equation that equals effective diagnosis and management. But what personalities are best? What are the necessary interpersonal relations that go into effective clinical operations? To begin, we must distinguish between the personality we *are* and the personality we *become* in the clinical setting. It has been said somewhere that we wear many masks for the different people we interact with. That is, we modify, to some degree, our interpersonal relations depending upon the person(s) we deal with. Consequently, different people may get different ideas or perceptions about our personalities.

We must realize that our *basic personality* may not be the reason we have clinical difficulties; however, our ability to play a role (personality) appropriate for the therapy setting may be less than adequate. We may not be putting on a wardrobe suitable to wear into the therapy room! And I am not talking about jeans versus a skirt or a T-shirt versus a shirt and tie. I am talking about the type of person you come across to your client as being while you are interacting with him or her in the clinical environment.

Now, it is also obvious that the larger discrepancy between your basic personality and your *clinical personality,* the more uncomfortable your clinical duties will become. However, who ever said that you should feel comfortable all the time? Aren't you entitled to your moments of unease and uncertainty? We said that certain clinical roles will facilitate therapeutic endeavors, but we did not say it would necessarily be easy or comfortable for you to enact those roles.

Your clinical personality should be as nonjudgmental as possible. You must become as sensitive a listener as possible, as objectively critical and at the same time appropriately reinforcing as you can be. You must convey belief that the person can and will change. You must convey an interest in the person as a person, and not just as a stutterer or as a set of interesting behaviors. Rogers' clinical tenet of *unconditional positive regard* is a good facet to add to your clinical personality. You must be able to open yourself up to client's questions, about who and what you are, but at the same time realize when you need to take charge and shift the focus of the therapy interaction. Above all, your personality must convey to the client a sincere interest in his or her welfare, without becoming emotionally involved to the point where your objectivity vanishes and your ability to assist the person diminishes.

Do you have to be outgoing to be a good clinician, or can you be the shy, retiring type and still be effective? This question is inappropriate. Let us see what you do in the clinical setting. If you are continually cracking jokes to maintain attention, running off at the mouth, and being in general a hail-fellow-well-met, but giving clients no indication that you care about them or their problems, your clinical personality is inappropriate. Clients are apt to say of such clinicians, "Well, he's a nice person, but I don't think he understands me and my problem." On the other hand, if you religiously run through your clinical exercises, give minimal exposure to your personal frailities, and are basically standoffish, then you have problems. Of these clincians clients usually say "They seem to know about my problems, but they really don't care about me, the person." In essence, your clinical personality, whatever its form (and this form may have to be changed depending upon the client or clinical setting), must convey and reflect

1. An interest in the client as a person;
2. A knowledge about the problem(s) at hand;
3. Ability to assist the client in making change and belief that such change is possible;
4. Objective assessment of behaviors, situations, and personal variables and minimal judgmental statements;
5. Sensitivity towards the client's, and your's, involvement in the human condition first and his or her problem(s) second.

the development of a clinician: from classroom to clinic

We take courses (short and long), sit through endless lectures, participate in seminars, and involve ourselves in independent studies. Our education is long and demanding. And then, one day, we step into the clinic for our first diagnostic or therapy session.

Suddenly, it seems, we are in another realm. We face a different world of real people with real problems who want our help and guidance and comfort. Gone are the books discussing hypothesis A versus hypothesis B. No more do we engage in the fascinating seminar discussions of whether a particular problem is learned or innate. We are on the line with a client, and time must be spent in a professional way. The way we spend this time, however, is the crux of our professional abilities.

Not all information we achieve in our education is readily applicable to the clinical process. This does not mean the information is useless, but sometimes clinicians express this opinion. What they appear to fail to realize is that education develops particular thought processes as well as it provides specific course content. Instead of accepting black or white approaches to the world, education tells us that many events are situated along a continuum. Such a relativistic notion does not excuse clinicians from making decisions; however, it should influence the type of decisions they make. Similarly, education instructs that problem solving, which asks answerable questions, tests them, and rejects and/or accepts hypotheses on the basis of findings is more appropriate than waiting for the answer from the expert(s).

Education expands horizons and our abilities to deal with change; it does not simply fill empty vessels. Surely, you cannot think in a vacuum—no one expects you to deal with communicative disorders without certain basic facts, figures, information, and concepts, but somewhere along the way, it is up to you to bridge the gap between classroom and clinic.

We often hear the claim, by clinicians in trouble, "If-I'd-only-had-so-and-so-in-such-and-such-course-then-I'd-be-all-right." The truth is however, that these clinicians are not applying even the limited amount of information they do have! They appear to see no relation between that which they learned and that which they must do in the clinic. They seem to expect the clinical process to take care of itself ("All I need is experience"). Experience, in and of itself, will lead them nowhere if the experience does not involve their active participation. Practice does not make perfect. Perfect practice makes perfect.

Student-clinicians having trouble in the clinic do not seem able to transfer from the academic to clinical setting. This lack of transference may result from a number of things: They did not really learn the content of their courses, (classroom excellence is often reflected in clinical excellence) or they did not really change their thought processes as a result of their education (they are still waiting around to be shown how to do it).

Many times such clinicians seem unable to compartmentalize their personal from their professional lives. Problems at home creep into and interfere with their clinical performance. "I couldn't concentrate on therapy because I'm worried about getting my car fixed."

Problem student-clinicians avoid evaluations of their supervisors and professors with the claim, "I tried to reach you but you weren't in." Interestingly, student-clinicians *without* clinical concerns always seem to find their supervisors and professors in their office. The less than adequate student-clinician claims, "No one told me I was doing poorly." Perhaps, this is so, but often they were told and they did not hear or listen. Short of being told, "We are flunking you out," problem student-clinicians do not seem to understand their supervisors when they say there are concerns or problems with the student's performance. Such students appear to lack the ability to self-analyze and to receive and act upon objective criticism they receive from their supervisors and professors.

A really unfortunate situation arises when student-clinicians, who have received negative objective evaluations of their clinical performance, begin to overly rely on supervisor-professor input for their clinical endeavors. They seem to be looking to some big person for help because they have received negative evaluation, and they become tremendously unsure of how to proceed. This fosters a vicious cycle where supervisors begin to see clinicians as overly dependent on feedback for clinical performance. Student-clinicians, in turn, come to overly rely on this feedback and do not develop their ability to independently problem solve and perform. Such cycles are difficult to break once started; we need to be aware of their potential for development so that we can head off their very existence.

Looking to others for assistance and suggestions is reasonable and appropriate, but when it becomes routine and habitual, it has the real potential for thwarting personal growth and independence. Self-responsibility for our lives, while never easy, is an absolute must for the development of an independent clinician. We all lapse back into stages of dependence, but hopefully we pick ourselves up off the floor and try to regain self-responsibility for our acts. It is our responsibility to apply course content to clinical endeavor. We must be the person to employ the necessary problem-solving orientation to the clinical situation. An active role is needed on the part of the clinician, and passivity will result in little change and growth. Although it may be a comfort to blame external factors for our inabilities, in the long run, it is we ourselves who must come to grips with the demands of the clinical interaction and try to rise to the challenge.

Self-analysis, problem solving, dedication to the task at hand, independence of thought and action, creative reactions to new situations, and the ability to transfer information from class to clinic are some of the more important hallmarks of a good student-clinician. Although very few people achieve all of these hallmarks to the ideal degree, many people are working to achieve such goals. They are at least aware of the presence of these goals and believe them to be of importance. We can become all the clinician we can become as long as we realize that we are the ones who have to do the becoming.

how much training you have had

There is great temptation to get defensive when a patient or client asks you how much training you have had. There are times when we do not like people poking around into our professional credentials. How we handle such questions, however, reflects as much on our training as it does on our maturity, experience, and so forth.

First, if at all possible, find out why you are being so questioned. Maybe you say to the person, "I understand your interest, but why do you ask?" In any case, try to find out why you are being questioned about your credentials. Sometimes clients are shopping around for the best (in their opinion) clinician, and other times they are simply testing you. It is important to distinguish between the two motivations.

Secondly, look to yourself. What signals are you giving that elicit such a question? Is it your apparent uncertainty, or is it your lack of ease with a client or what? Remember to keep in mind the difference between your uncertainty as a clinician-person and your uncertainty regarding the handling of a particularly unique, difficult, or unclear case. If you are young (especially your physical appearance and manner of expression), you can just expect more queries about your credentials or experiences. There is no need to get defensive. Remember, experience comes from going through the experiences you are going through.

Finally, have your past successes (or lack thereof) with a particular age client, parents, or communicative disorders finally caught up with you?

Perhaps, if time or money permits, a course in the area of concern (no matter if you have had a course with the same title or not) may be a wise investment. We are never, thank goodness, too old to learn or relearn. If nothing else, start picking up books and journals and read.

"my child's been with *you* for three months and I don't see any change"

Lack of progress, or no apparent new behavior, is often the beginning of the end of a therapy program. Parents who do not see any progress become less likely to chauffeur little Johnny in for his twice-a-week therapy. Johnny, likewise, is apt to become frustrated, less willing to work, and less motivated if he detects lack of progress, and the clinician, poor person, becomes depressed at the living testimony to his or her ineptness.

Surely, one does not want to whitewash incompetent methods which have resulted in minimal clinical progress. Likewise, one does not want to excuse the reluctant client and his or her parents who will not or cannot cooperate in the therapy process to bring about a change. We must, however, realize when lack of progress is really telling us something about the problem(s) we are dealing with.

First, have we evaluated and diagnosed the situation correctly and completely? Are we ignoring some important variable, for example, a limited attention span, because we believe the client can rise above such trivia and exert enough will power to improve. Therapy, it has been said, is a continual diagnostic experience; however, many times we forget this in the rush to fill the therapy hour with methods to effect the cure.

Secondly, does lack of progress really indicate that perhaps we are expecting change prior to change being possible? Are we becoming unnecessarily anxious with the slowness of the behavioral change process? Parents, particularly, are susceptible to wanting to speed up the pace of their child's development. Parents give us important cues to this when they tell us that Billy's stuttering ". . . is holding him back and if he can lick this thing he'll be able to do much . . . he has so much potential . . . he's got to change it now before it's too late." They become impatient with our procedures, especially when those procedures do not work on his speech. Clearly, it is our role to tell parents, from the beginning, approximately how long therapy will take and what steps it will involve. Children must crawl before they walk, and parents must be made to understand this. No matter how much they love their child and desire for their child's well-being, the learning process cannot be sped up. There are no free lunches.

Thirdly, clients may become depressed at the rate of progress because they envisioned you as the guru who was going to lift the stuttering burden off their shoulders without any sweat, pain, work, and travail on their part. It comes as a surprise to them when they learn that behavioral changes require them to work and practice every day at changing their speech. What is wrong, they think; it is not supposed to be this hard. I thought this speech doctor was supposed to cure me. Some doctor!

The client, like the impatient parent, must realize that change takes time, work, and patience. The longest journey begins with a single step and all that. We, as clinicians, must clearly articulate to the clients our goals and subgoals and the time frame within such goals will be realized. We must set our clients up for the inevitable wall of inertia they will meet when they begin to try to change their old, well-learned, but inappropriate, behavior. If we expect more stuttering before less stuttering, we should tell the client and the parents. We might explain that for change to occur, the client must diminish his or her circumlocutions and avoidances and actually stutter. Likewise, we should tell the client and parents what they might look for in terms of signs of early improvement, for example, decreased duration of stutterings.

Even the most seemingly depressing situation like that of a no progress client is an opportunity for developing our clinical skills and assisting our client. Asking questions with regard to the whys of the no progress evaluation will provide the opportunity. Looking for answers from the experts and books will provide us some assistance, but we may maximize the potential of the opportunity. Our progress as clinicians, like that of our clients, has a certain price, but fortunately all of us have the potential to pay this price. Some of us just think we are paupers or that there is a bargain basement.

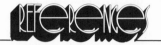

ADAMS, M. A., "A Physiologic and Aerodynamic Interpretation of Fluent and Stuttered Speech," *Journal of Fluency Disorders*, 4, 78–89 (1974).

ADAMS, M. A., "A Clinical Strategy for Differentiating the Normally Nonfluent Child and the Incipient Stutterer," *Journal of Fluency Disorders*, 2, 141–148 (1977).

ADAMS, M., and P. HAYDEN, "The Ability of Stutterers and Nonstutterers to Initiate and Terminate Phonation During Production of an Isolated Vowel," *Journal of Speech Hearing Research*, 19, 290–296 (1976).

ADAMS, M., and P. RAMIG, "Vocal Characteristics of Normal Speakers and Stutterers during Choral Reading," *Journal of Speech Hearing Research*, 23, 457–469 (1980).

AINSWORTH, S. (ed.), *If Your Child Stutters: A Guide for Parents.* Memphis, Tenn.: Speech Foundation of America, 1977.

AMMONS, R., and R. AMMONS, "The Quick Test (QT): Provisional Manual," *Psychological Reports*, 11, 111–161 (1962) (Monogr. Suppl. I–VII).

ANDREWS, G., and M. HARRIS, *The Syndrome of Stuttering.* London: Heinemann Medical Books, 1964.

AXLINE, V. M., *Play Therapy.* Boston: Houghton Mifflin, 1947.

BATES, E., "Pragmatics and Sociolinguistics in Child Language," in *Normal and Deficient Child Language*, eds. D. Morehead and A. Morehead. Baltimore: University Park Press, 1976.

BEECH, H., and F. FRANSELLA, *Research and Experiment in Stuttering.* Oxford England: Pergamon Press, 1968.

BEECHER, H. K., "The Powerful Placebo," *Journal American Medical Association*, 159, 1602–1606 (1955).

BENSON, H., *The Relaxation Response.* New York: Avon Books, 1976.

BENSON, H., and M. D., EPSTEIN, "The Placebo Effect: A Neglected Asset in the Care of Patients," *Journal of American Medical Association*, 232, 1225–1227 (1975).

BENSON, H., and D. McCALLIE, "Angina Pectoris and the Placebo Effect," *New England Journal of Medicine*, 300, 1424–1429 (1979).

BINGHAM, J., *Courage to Change: An Introduction to the Life and Thought of Reinhold Niebuhr.* Boston: Little, Brown, 1961.

BLOODSTEIN, O., "The Development of Stuttering: I. Changes in Nine Basic Features," *Journal of Speech Hearing Disorders*, 25, 219–237 (1960a)

BLOODSTEIN, O., "The Development of Stuttering: II. Developmental Phases," *Journal of Speech Hearing Disorders*, 25, 366–376 (1960b).

BLOODSTEIN, O., "The Development of Stuttering: III. Developmental Phases," *Journal of Speech Hearing Disorders*, 26, 67–82 (1961).

BLOODSTEIN, O., *A Handbook on Stuttering.* Chicago: National Easter Seal Society for Crippled Children and Adults, 1975a.

BLOODSTEIN, O., "Stuttering as Tension and Fragmentation," in *Stuttering: A Second Symposium,* ed. J. Eisenson. New York: Harper & Row, Pub. 1975b.

BOEHMLER, R., "Listener Responses to Non-Fluencies," *Journal of Speech Hearing Research,* 1, 132–141 (1958).

BOONE, O., *The Voice and Voice Therapy* (2nd ed.). Englewood Cliffs, N. J.: Prentice-Hall, Inc., 1977.

BRAYTON, E., and E. CONTURE, "Effects of Noise and Rhythmic Stimulation on the Speech of Stutterers." *Journal of Speech Hearing Research,* 21, 285–294 (1978).

BROWN, R., *A First Language/The Early Stages.* Cambridge, Mass.: Harvard University Press, 1973.

BRUTTEN, E., and D. SHOEMAKER, *The Modification of Stuttering.* Englewood Cliffs, N. J.: Prentice-Hall, Inc., 1967.

CARKHUFF, R. R., *The Art of Problem-Solving.* Amherst, Mass.: Human Resource Development Press, 1973.

CONTURE, E., "Some Effects of Noise on the Speaking Behavior of Stutterers," *Journal of Speech Hearing Research,* 17, 714–723 (1974).

CONTURE, E., and E. BRAYTON, "The Influence of Noise on Stutterers' Different Disfluency Types," *Journal of Speech Hearing Research,* 18, 381–384 (1975).

CONTURE, E., and A. CARUSO, "Book Review: The Stocker Probe Technique for Diagnosis and Treatment of Stuttering in Young Children (a test developed by Beatrice Stocker)," *Journal of Fluency Disorders,* 3, 297–298 (1978).

CONTURE, E., G. MCCALL, and D. BREWER, "Laryngeal Behavior during Stuttering," *Journal of Speech Hearing Research,* 20, 661–668 (1977).

CONTURE, E., and D. METZ, "The Influence of Rhythmic Stimulation on Certain Vocal Characteristics of Stutterers." A paper presented to the 14th Annual Convention of the New York State Speech and Hearing Association (1974).

CONTURE, E., and E. VAN NAERSSEN, "Reading Abilities of School-Age Stutterers," *Journal of Fluency Disorders,* 2, 295–300 (1977).

COOPER, E., "Intervention Procedures for the Young Stutterer," in *Controversies About Stuttering Therapy,* ed. H. Gregory. Baltimore: University Park Press, 1978.

COOPER, E., *Understanding Stuttering: Information for Parents.* Chicago: National Easter Seal Society for Crippled Children and Adults, 1979.

CROSS, D., and H. LUPER, "Voice Reaction Time of Stuttering and Nonstuttering Children and Adults," *Journal of Fluency Disorders,* 4, 59–77 (1979).

DALTON, P., and W. J. HARDCASTLE, *Disorders of Fluency.* New York: Elsevier, 1977.

DARLEY, F., A. ARONSON, and J. BROWN, *Motor Speech Disorders*. Philadelphia: Saunders, 1975.

DARLEY, F., and D. SPRIESTERSBACH, *Diagnostic Methods in Speech Pathology* (2nd ed.). New York: Harper & Row, Pub., 1978.

DAVIS, D. M., "The Relation of Repetitions in the Speech of Young Children to Measures of Language Maturity and Situational Factors: Part I," *Journal of Speech Disorders*, 4, 303–318 (1939).

DAVIS, D. M., "The Relation of Repetitions in the Speech of Young Children to Certain Measures of Language Maturity and Situational Factors: Part II & III," *Journal of Speech Disorders*, 5, 235–246 (1940).

DELL, C. W., *Treating the School Age Stutterer: A Guide for Clinicians*. Memphis, Tenn.: Speech Foundation of America, 1980.

DODSON, F., *How to Parent*. New York: Signet, 1970.

DOUGLASS, E., and R. QUARRINGTON, "The Differentiation of Interiorized and Exteriorized Secondary Stuttering," *Journal of Speech Hearing Disorders*, 17, 377–385 (1952).

FAIRCLOTH, S., and M. FAIRCLOTH, *Phonetic Science: A Program of Instruction*. Englewood Cliffs, N. J.: Prentice-Hall, Inc., 1973.

FOURCIN, A., "Laryngograph Examination of the Vocal Fold Vibration," in *Ventilatory and Phonatory Control Mechanisms*, ed. B. Wyke. Oxford, England: Oxford University Press, 1974, pp. 315–333.

FOURCIN, A., "Larynogographic Assessment of Phonatory Function." Proceedings of Conference on Assessment of Vocal Fold Pathology, National Institute of Health, Bethesda, Maryland (April 17 and 18, 1979; to be published).

FREEMAN, F., "Phonation in Stuttering: A Review of Current Research," *Journal of Fluency Disorders*, 4, 79–89 (1979).

FREEMAN, F., and T. USHIJIMA, "Laryngeal Muscle Activity during Stuttering," *Journal of Speech Hearing Research*, 21, 538–562 (1978).

GINOTT, H., *Between Parent and Teenager*. New York: Avon, 1969.

GREGORY, H., *Stuttering: Differential Evaluation and Therapy*. Indianapolis: Bobbs-Merrill, 1973.

GREGORY, H., (ed.), *Controversies about Stuttering Therapy*. Baltimore: University Park Press, 1978.

GUITAR, B., "Reduction of Stuttering Frequency Using Analog Electro–Myographic Feedback," *Journal of Speech Hearing Research*, 18, 672–685 (1975).

GUITAR, B., M. ADAMS, and E. CONTURE, "Clinical Feedback," *Journal of Childhood Communication Disorders*, 3, 3–12 (1979).

GUITAR, B., and T. PETERS, *Stuttering: An Integration of Contemporary Therapies*. Memphis, Tenn.: Speech Foundation of America, 1980.

GUYTON, A., *Textbook of Medical Physiology*, (4th ed.). Philadelphia: Saunders, 1971.

HALL, H., *Help Wanted?: A Guidebook for Parents and Therapist Dealing with Young Nonfluent Children*. Evanston, Ill.: Junior League of Evanston, Inc., 1966.

HARDY, J., "Development of Neuromuscular Systems Underlying Speech Production," in *Speech and the Dentofacial Complex: The State of the Art, ASHA Reports,* 5, 49–68 (1970).

HARDY, J. "Basic Concepts — Neural Processes of Speech and Language," in *Processes and Disorders of Human Communication,* ed. J. Curtis. New York: Harper & Row, Pub., 1978.

HARRIS, T., *I'm OK—You're OK.* New York: Harper & Row, Pub., 1967.

HILL, W. F., *Learning: A Survey of Psychological Interpretations* (3rd ed.). New York: Harper & Row, Pub., 1977.

HILLMAN, R., and H. GILBERT, "Voice Onset Time for Voiceless Stop Consonants in the Fluent Reading of Stutterers and NonStutterers," *Journal Acoustical Society of America,* 61, 610–611 (1977).

HUFFMAN, E., and W. PERKINS, "Dysfluency Characteristics Identified by Listeners as 'Stuttering' and 'Stutterer,' " *Journal of Communicative Diseases,* 7, 89–96 (1974).

HUTCHINSON, J., "Aerodynamic Patterns of Stuttered Speech," in *Vocal Tract Dynamics and Disfluency,* eds. M. Webster and L. Furst. New York: Speech and Hearing Institute of New York, 1974, pp. 71–123.

ILG, F., and L. AMES, *Child Behavior.* New York: Dell Pub., Co., Inc., 1960.

JOHNSON, W., *People in Quandries.* New York: Harper & Row, Pub., 1946.

JOHNSON, W., "An Open Letter to the Mother of a Stuttering Child," *Journal of Speech Hearing Disorders,* 14, 3–8 (1949).

JOHNSON, W., *Stuttering and What You Can Do About It.* Minneapolis, Minn.: University of Minnesota Press, 1961.

JOHNSON, W., F. DARLEY, and D. SPRIESTERSBACH, *Diagnostic Methods in Speech Pathology.* New York: Harper & Row, Pub., 1963.

JOHNSON, W., and OTHERS, *The Onset of Stuttering.* Minneapolis, Minn.: University of Minnesota Press, 1959.

JOHNSON, W., and OTHERS, *Speech Handicapped School Children* (3rd Ed.). New York: Harper & Row, Pub., 1967.

JOHNSTON, J., and T. SCHERY, "The Use of Grammatical Morphemes by Children with Communication Disorders," in *Normal and Deficient Child Language,* eds. E. Morehead and A. Morehead. Baltimore: University Park Press, 1976.

KIDD, K., and OTHERS, "A Genetic Perspective on Stuttering," *Journal of Fluency Disorders,* 4, 259–270 (1977).

KIRITANI, S., "Articulatory Studies by the X-Ray Microbeam System," in *Dynamic Aspects of Speech,* eds. M. Sawashima and E. Cooper. Tokyo, Japan: University of Tokyo Press, 1977.

KLATT, D., "Voice Onset Time, Frication and Aspiration in Word-Initial Consonant Clusters," *Journal of Speech Hearing Research,* 18, 686–706 (1975).

LEFRANCOIS, G., *Psychological Theories and Human Learning: Kongor's Report.* Monterey, Calif.: Brooks/Cole, 1972.

LE SHAN, E., *How to Survive Parenthood.* New York: Warner Paperback Library, 1963.

LUPER, H., and R. MULDER, *Stuttering Therapy for Children.* Englewood Cliffs, N. J.: Prentice-Hall, Inc., 1964.

McDONALD, E., *Articulation Testing and Treatment: A Sensory-Motor Approach.* Pittsburgh: Stanwix House, Inc., 1964.

MASTERS, W., and V. JOHNSON, *Human Sexual Inadequacy.* New York: Little, Brown, 1970.

METZ, D., E. CONTURE, and A. CARUSO, "Voice Onset Time, Frication and Aspiration during Stutterers' Fluent Speech," *Journal of Speech Hearing Research,* 22, 649–656 (1979).

METZ, D., J. ONUFRAK, and R. S. OGBURN, "An Acoustical Analysis of Stutterer's Speech Prior to and at the Termination of Therapy," *Journal of Fluency Disorders,* 4, 249–254 (1979).

MILLER, N., "Experimental Studies of Conflict," in *Personality and the Behavior Disorders,* ed. J. Hunt. New York: Ronald Press, 1944.

MURPHY, A., and R. FITZSIMONS, *Stuttering and Personality Dynamics.* New York: Ronald Press, 1960.

NEILL, A., *Summerhill: A Radical Approach to Child Rearing.* New York: Hart Associates, 1960.

NETSELL, R., "Speech Physiology," in *Normal Aspects of Speech, Hearing and Language,* eds. R. Minifie, T. Hixon, and F. Williams. Englewood Cliffs, N. J.: Prentice-Hall, Inc., 1973.

NIEBUHR, R., "Prayer" (1934), in *Bartlett's Familiar Quotations,* (14th ed.), ed. E. M. Beck. Boston: Little, Brown, 1968.

PERKINS, W. H., "Physiological Studies," in *Stuttering: Research Therapy,* ed. J. G. Sheehan. New York: Harper & Row, Pub., 1970.

PERKINS, W. H., "From Psychoanalysis to Discoordination," in *Controversies About Stuttering Therapy,* ed. H. H. Gregory. Baltimore: University Park Press, 1978.

PERKINS, W. H., "Disorders of Speech Flow," in *Introduction to Communication Disorders,* eds. T. Hixon, L. Shriberg, and J. Saxman. Englewood Cliffs, N. J.: Prentice-Hall, Inc., 1980.

PERKINS, W., and others, "Stuttering: Discoordination of Phonation with Articulation and Respiration," *Journal of Speech Hearing Research,* 19, 509–522 (1976).

PRINS, D., "Motivation/Part One," in *Therapy for Stutterers,* ed. C. Starkweather. Memphis, Tenn.: Speech Foundation of Amercia, 1974.

REES, N., "Learning to Talk and Understand," in *Introduction to Communicative Disorders,* eds. T. Hixon, L. Shriberg, and J. Saxman. Englewood Cliffs, N. J.: Prentice-Hall, Inc., 1980.

REYNOLDS, G., *A Primer of Operant Conditioning.* Glenview, Ill.: Scott, Foresman, 1968.

RIEBER, R. W. (ed.), *The Problem of Stuttering: Theory and Therapy.* New York: Elsevier (1977).

ROBINSON, F., *Introduction to Stuttering.* Englewood Cliffs, N. J.: Prentice-Hall, Inc., 1964.

ROSENBEK, J., and OTHERS, "Stuttering Following Brain Damage," *Brain and Language*, 6, 82–96 (1978).

ROTHENBERG, M., "Some Relations between Glottal Airflow and Vocal Fold Contact Area." Proceedings of the Conference on the Assessment of Vocal Pathology, National Institutes of Health, Bethesda, Maryland (April 17 and 18, 1979; to be published).

RUNYAN, C., and M. ADAMS, "Perceptual Study of 'Successfully Therapeuterized' Stutterers," *Journal of Fluency Disorders*, 3, 25–39 (1978).

RYAN, B. "Stuttering Therapy in a Framework of Operant Conditioning and Programmed Learning," in *Controversies About Stuttering Therapy*, ed. H. Gregory. Baltimore: University Park Press, 1978.

SCHWARTZ, M. F., *Stuttering Solved.* Philadelphia: Lippincott, 1976.

SEEBACH, M., and A. CARUSO, "Voice Onset Time during the Fluent Speech of Young Stutterers." Paper presented at Annual Convention of the American Speech and Hearing Association, Atlanta, Georgia (1979).

SHAEFER, C. E., "Raising Children by Old-Fashioned Parent Sense," *Children Today* (A publication of the Children's Bureau, ACYF, DHEW [November–December, 1978]).

SHAMES, G., and D. EGOLF, *Operant Conditioning and the Management of Stuttering*, Englewood Cliffs, N. J.: Prentice-Hall, Inc., 1976.

SHAMES, G., and C. FLORANCE, *Stutter-Free Speech: A Goal for Therapy.* Columbus, Ohio: Chas. E. Merrill, 1980.

SHAPIRO, A., "Factors Contributing to the Placebo Effect: Their Implications for Psychotherapy," *American Journal of Psychotherapy*, 18, Suppl. 1, 73–88 (1964).

SHAPIRO, A., "An Electromyographic Analysis of the Fluent and Dysfluent Utterances of Several Types of Stutterers," *Journal of Fluency Disorders*, 5, 203–231 (1980).

SHEEHAN, J., "Conflict Theory of Stuttering," in *Stuttering: A Symposium*, ed. J. Eisenson. New York: Harper & Row, Pub., 1958.

SHEEHAN, J., "Reflections on the Behavioral Modification of Stuttering," in *Conditioning in Stuttering Therapy*, ed. C. Starkweather. Memphis, Tenn.: Speech Foundation of America, 1970a.

SHEEHAN, J., "Personality Approaches," in *Stuttering: Research and Therapy*, ed. J. G. Sheehan. New York: Harper & Row, Pub., 1970b.

SHEEHAN, J., "Conflict Theory and Avoidance-Reduction Therapy," in *Stuttering: A Second Symposium*, ed. J. Eisenson. New York: Harper & Row, Pub., 1975.

SHEEHAN, J., "Current Issues on Stuttering and Recovery," in *Controversies About Stuttering Therapy*, ed. H. Gregory. Baltimore: University Park Press, 1978.

SHRIBERG, L., and OTHERS, "The Wisconsin Procedure for Appraisal of Clinical Competence (W–PACC): Model and Data," *ASHA*, 17, 158–165 (1975).

SHRIBERG, L., and J. KWIATKOWSKI, *Natural Process Analysis (NPA): A Procedure for Phonological Analyses of Continuous Speech Samples.* Baltimore: University Park Press, 1980.

SIEGEL, G., "Punishment, Stuttering and Disfluency," *Journal of Speech Hearing Research*, 13, 677–714 (1970).

SKINNER, B. F., *Science and Human Behavior*. New York: Macmillan, 1953.

SKOLNICK, M. L., and G. N. McCALL, "Velopharyngeal Competence and Incompetence Following Pharyngeal Flap Surgery; A Video-Fluroscopic Study in Multiple Projections," *Cleft Palate Journal*, 9 (1972).

SPOCK, B., *Pocketbook of Baby and Child Care*. New York: Pocket Books, 1946.

STARBUCK, H., "Motivation/Part Two," in *Therapy for Stutterers*, ed. C. Starkweather. Memphis, Tenn.: Speech Foundation of America, 1974.

STARKWEATHER, C. (ed.), *Therapy for Stutterers*. Memphis, Tenn.: Speech Foundation of America, 1974.

STEVENS, K., D. KALIKOW, and T. WILLEMAIN, "Research Note: A Miniature Accelerometer for Detecting Glottal Waveforms and Nasalization," *Journal of Speech Hearing Research*, 18, 594–599 (1979).

STOCKER, B., *Stocker Probe Technique for Diagnosis and Treatment of Stuttering in Young Children*. Tulsa, Oklahoma: Modern Education Corporation, 1976.

STROMSTA, C., and S. FIBIGER, "Physiological Correlates of the Core Behavior of Stuttering." Paper presented to XVIIIth *IALP Congress*, Washington, D.C. (1980).

TURNER, P., *Clinical Aspects of Autonomic Pharmacology*. Philadelphia: Lippincott, 1969.

VAILLANT, G., *Adaptation to Life*. Boston: Little, Brown, 1977.

VAN RIPER, C., "Historical Approaches," in *Stuttering: Research and Therapy*, ed. J. Sheehan. New York: Harper & Row, Pub., 1970.

VAN RIPER, C., *The Nature of Stuttering*. Englewood Cliffs, N. J.: Prentice-Hall, Inc., 1971.

VAN RIPER, C., *The Treatment of Stuttering*. Englewood Cliffs, N. J.: Prentice-Hall, Inc., 1973.

VAN RIPER, C., "Modification of Behavior," in *Therapy for Stutterers*, ed. C. Starkweather. Memphis, Tenn.: Speech Foundation of America, 1974.

VAN RIPER, C., "The Stutterer's Clinician," in *Stuttering: A Second Symposium*, ed. J. Eisenson. New York: Harper & Row, Pub., 1975.

WEBSTER, R., *The Precision Fluency Shaping Program: Clinician's Program Guide*. Blacksburg, Virginia: University Publications, 1975.

WEBSTER, R., "Empirical Considerations Regarding Stuttering Therapy," in *Controversies About Stuttering Therapy*, ed. H. Gregory. Baltimore: University Park Press, 1978.

WILLIAMS, D. E., "A Point of View About 'Stuttering,' " *Journal of Speech Hearing Disorders*, 22, 390–397 (1957).

WILLIAMS, D. E., "Stuttering Therapy: an Overview," in *Learning Theory and Stuttering Therapy*, ed. H. Gregory. Evanston, Ill.: Northwestern University Press, 1968.

WILLIAMS, D. E., "Stuttering Therapy for Children," in *Handbook of Speech Pathology and Audiology*, ed. L. E. Travis. Englewood Cliffs, N. J.: Prentice-Hall, Inc., 1971.

WILLIAMS, D. E., "Evaluation," in *Therapy for Stutterers*, ed. C. Starkweather. Memphis, Tenn.: Speech Foundation of America, 1974.

WILLIAMS, D. E., "A Perspective on Approaches to Stuttering Therapy," in *Controversies About Stuttering Therapy*, ed. H. Gregory. Baltimore: University Park Press, 1978.

WILLIAMS, D., and L. KENT, "Listener Evaluations of Speech Interruptions," *Journal of Speech Hearing Research*, 1, 124–131 (1958).

WILLIAMS, D., F. SILVERMAN, and J. KOOLS, "Disfluency Behavior of Elementary-School Age Stutterers and Nonstutterers: Loci of Instances of Disfluency," *Journal of Speech Hearing Research*, 12, 308–318 (1969).

WINGATE, M. E., "A Standard Definition of Stuttering," *Journal of Speech Hearing Disorders*, 29, 484–489 (1964).

WINGATE, M. E., "Sound and Pattern in 'Artificial' Fluency," *Journal of Speech Hearing Research*, 12, 677–686 (1969).

WINGATE, M. E., "The Fear of Stuttering," *ASHA*, 13, 3–5 (1971).

WINGATE, M. E., *Stuttering Theory and Treatment*. New York: Irvington Publishers, 1976.

WINITZ, H., "Repetitions in the Vocalizations of Children in the First Two Years of Life," *Journal of Speech Hearing Disorders*, Monogra Supplies, 7, 55–62 (1961).

WINITZ, H., *Articulatory Acquisition and Behavior*. Englewood Cliffs, N. J.: Prentice-Hall, Inc., 1969.

WINN, M., *The Plug-In Drug*. New York: Viking, 1977.

YAIRI, E., and N. F. CLIFTON, JR., "Disfluent Speech Behavior of Preschool Children, High School Seniors, and Geriatric Persons," *Journal of Speech Hearing Research*, 15, 714–719 (1972).

ZILBERGELD, B., and M. EVENS, "The Inadequacy of Masters and Johnson," *Psychology Today*, 14, 28–43 (1980).

ZIMMERMAN, G., "Articulatory Dynamics of Fluent Utterances of Stutterers and Nonstutterers," *Journal of Speech Hearing Research*, 23, 95–107 (1980a).

ZIMMERMAN, G., "Articulatory Behaviors Associated with Stuttering: A Cinefluorographic Analysis," *Journal of Speech Hearing Research*, 23, 108–121 (1980b).

ZWITMAN, D., *The Disfluent Child*. Baltimore: University Park Press, 1978.

Aberrancies, as pre-stuttering behavior, 12
Academic problems, conflict with therapy, 33, 102
Acting out, 77, 103
Adams, M., 31, 83, 145, 146, 151
Adams, M.A., 3, 37, 61
Adjustment problems, 3
Adolescence, 90–91
Adolescent:
    attitudes towards therapy, 70, 91
    concerns of, 101–5
    psychosocial problems of, 90–91, 99
    therapy procedures, 90–106
Adolescent-adult interaction, 91
Adult:
    therapy procedures, 109–37
    therapy referral, 37–38
    voice onset time, 31
Aerodynamic back pressure, 57
Age:
    chronological, 32
    relation to language disorders, 17, 27, 29, 33, 42, 44, 45
Ainsworth, S., 10, 12, 15, 37, 44, 45, 54, 79, 163
Alpha stage, of stuttering, 12, 13, 14
Ames, L., 47
Ammons, R., 35
Ammon's Quick Test, 48
Analogies:
    of sound transition, 62–63
    of speech production, 56–60, 84, 98, 123, 132
Andrews, G., 42, 127
Anticipation, of stuttering, 10
Anxiety, 80
Apraxic disorders, 110
Aronson, A., 30, 35, 110, 118
Articulation, 30–31, 32, 48, 49, 121 *See also* Speech
Articulatory contact, 9, 146
Attitudes:
    towards stuttering, 9, 108–9
    towards therapist, 20
    towards therapy, 63–64, 70, 79, 111
Auditory sensitivity-discrimination, 30
Awareness, 10, 26, 47, 54, 71, 72–74, 120, 131, 141

objective, 73, 83
subjective, 73–74
Axline, V. M., 46

Barbs. *See* Disrupter, speech fluency
Bates, E., 52
Beech, H., 109
Beecher, H. K., 87
Behavioral description, 3, 13
Behavioral modification, 110, 142, 143–44
Behavior composite, 3, 8, 13, 29–30, 81–82, 134
Benson, H., 64, 87, 101
Beta Stage, of stuttering, 12, 13, 14
Bingham, J., 152
Biofeedback, 83
Bloodstein, O., 7, 8, 28, 29, 49, 80, 102, 146
Body movement, 8–11, 16, 29–30, 82
Body posture, 10
Body rigidity, 30
Boehmlee, R., 11
Boone, O., 30
Brain damage, 110
Brayton, E., 145, 146, 147
Brewer, D., 12, 31, 61, 83, 96
Brown, J., 30, 35, 110, 118
Brown, R., 47
Brutten, E., 9, 23, 59, 81

Carkhuff, R. R., 6
Caruso, A., 12, 31, 51, 97
Child:
    articulation in, 32
    awareness of stuttering, 47, 54, 71, 72–74
    comprehension of stuttering, 56, 61
    evaluation, 44–60
    readiness for therapy, 49–50
    therapy procedures, 40–68
    therapy referral, 37
    voice onset time, 30
Child development, 45, 77
Child-family counseling, 45, 99
Circumlocution, 80
Client. *See also* Stutterer
    beliefs and expectations, 87, 131–32
    identification information, 22–23
Clifton, N. F., Jr., 16

Clinician. *See* Speech-language pathologist
Closure, of speech mechanism, 57
Cognitive development, 16, 51
Communication, child-parent, 77–78
Communication media, influence on
    language development, 16
Communicative skill, age-related, 29
Contraction:
    nonspeech musculature, 8–11
    speech musculature, 8–11, 57, 83–84,
    124
Contraindications of therapy, 32, 44, 104
Conture, E., 12, 31, 33, 51, 61, 83, 96, 97,
    145, 146, 147
Conversation:
    interruption, 52, 76
    low-level, 51
Cooper, E., 44, 45, 65, 163
Counseling:
    child-family, 45
    parental, 15, 18, 32, 37, 43, 44–47,
    65–67, 85
    specialized, 108
Credentials, of therapist, 169–70
Credibility, of therapist, 46
Cross, D., 31
Cure, possibility of, 2, 113, 145, 151–52
Cyclic variation, 27, 47

Dalton, P., 150
Darley, F., 10, 30, 35, 110, 118
Davis, D. M., 16
Delay, of language development, 48, 104
Dell, C. W., 49
Delta stage, of stuttering, 14
Demonstration:
    of speech production, 60–61, 84, 96–98,
    126, 129
    of stuttering, 115, 118, 141
Denial, 36
Desensitization, 74–76, 77, 81, 130
Developmental stages, of stuttering, 11–14,
    80, 124
Diagnosis, 3, 6, 15–17 *See also* Evaluation
Diagnosogenic model, 162
Discontinuation, of therapy, 63–64, 86–87,
    92, 133–34
Disruptor, speech fluency, 74–77
Dodson, F., 47, 53
Douglass, E., 16, 92
Duration:
    of stuttering, 120, 121
    of therapy, 113–14

Egolf, D., 82, 91
Emotional discomfort, 10, 80, 87–88
Emotionality, 108, 109, 115, 122

Empathy, 148–50
Employer, referral by, 110
Employment capabilities, 20, 102–3
Environment, modification of, 18, 67
Epstein, M. D., 87
Equipment:
    for demonstrating speech production,
    60–61, 96–98
    for demonstrating stuttering, 115, 118,
    141
    for evaluating stuttering, 21–22, 141
    for speech practice, 99, 100–101
Etiology, of stuttering, 27–28, 144, 146,
    147–48
Evaluation, 8, 20–39, 42
    of adult, 108, 109–10
    of child, 44–60, 83
    importance of, 139–40
    of therapeutic progress, 101
Evaluation room, 21
Evens, M., 144
Eye contact, avoidance of, 10, 14, 37, 38,
    54, 79

Facial grimace, 55, 82
Faircloth, M., 143
Faircloth, S., 143
Fatigue, 30, 33
Fibiger, S., 12
Fitzsimons, R., 46
Florance, C., 145, 147
Fourcin, A., 98
Fransella, F., 109
Freeman, F., 3, 12, 31, 61, 83
Frequency:
    of stuttering, 133
    of therapy, 113–14
Fricative, misarticulation, 32
Frustration threshold, 74, 76

Gamma stage, of stuttering, 12, 13, 14, 124
Genetic basis, of stuttering, 46
Gestures, during speaking, 29, 30
Gilbert, H., 31
Ginott, H., 93, 98
Glide, misarticulation, 32
Gregory, H., 114, 147
Group norm, of speech disfluency, 16, 29
Group therapy, 38, 110–12, 115, 130
Guilt:
    of parents, 40, 48, 66
    of therapist, 121
Guitar, B., 28, 83, 147
Guyton, A., 59

Habituation, 92–93, 108, 131, 132, 144
Hall, H., 74, 77
Hardcastle, W. J., 150

Hardy, J., 35
Harris, M., 42, 127, 148
Hayden, P., 31
Head movements, 9, 29, 82
Hearing disorders, 30
Hill, W. F., 3
Hillman, R., 31
Homework, 63, 89–90, 112, 131
Huffman, E., 10
Hutchinson, J., 83
Hypnotherapy, 108

Identification, of stuttering occurrence,
    81–82, 114–22, 141
Identification information, on client, 22–23
Ilg, F., 47
Imitation, of therapist, 60, 81–82
Index, of stuttering, 21
Individuality, 4–5, 7, 15–16, 33, 35, 107
Individual therapy. See Therapy
Infection, middle-ear, 30
Informed consent, 22
Intake form, for evaluation, 22–23
Intelligence:
    individual variability, 20
    and therapeutic progress, 5, 33, 35
Interaction:
    adolescent-adult, 91
    parent-child, 46, 47, 50, 77–78
    with peers, 78, 103
    with sibling, 51–52, 53
Interpersonal skills:
    development of, 78
    of therapist, 20–21, 165–67
Interruption, of conversation, 51–52, 76
Interview procedure, 23–28, 154–57

"Job Task/Home Town" procedure, 101
Johnson, V., 144–45
Johnson, W., 3, 12, 25, 44, 89, 101, 122,
    158, 162
Johnston, J., 47

Kalikow, D., 26
Kent, L., 10, 11
Kidd, K., 46
Kiritani, S., 150
Kools, J., 16
Kwiatkowski, J., 32

Language development, 16, 51
    delayed, 48, 104
Language disorders, therapy for, 33
Laryngeal behavior, 31, 57, 150
    measurement, 96–97
Larynx closure, 57
Leader, of group therapy, 112
Learning disability (LD) specialist, 104

Learning process, 79
Lefrancois, G., 3
LeShan, E., 37, 41, 66
Lip closure, 57
Listener:
    differential responses, 10–11
    eye contact with, 10, 14, 37, 38, 54, 79,
        124
    perception of stuttering, 7–11, 18, 25–26
    reaction to stuttering, 73, 76
Listening to child, 76–77, 85
Luper, H., 31, 44

McCall, G., 12, 61, 83, 96
McCall, G. N., 26, 31
McCallie, D., 64, 87
McDonald, E., 32, 62
Master, W., 144–45
Maturity, of adolescent, 96
Mean length of utterance, 48, 120, 121
Metz, D., 31, 97, 146, 147, 151
Microcomputers, clinical applications, 6
Microscopic analysis, of speech behavior,
    22
Middle-ear infections, 30
Miller, N., 91
Mirrors, for speech practice, 60, 141
MLU. See Mean length of utterance
Model, speech, 54, 60, 88
Modification, 82–84, 92, 122–23
    automaticity of, 131–32
    beginning of, 121–22
    behavioral, 110, 142, 143–44
    reinforcement of, 127–28
    within therapy carryover, 128–30, 144
Monologues, 52, 53
Morpheme, 48, 121
Motion rate tasks, 35
Motivation, for therapy, 25, 35, 63–64, 70,
    80, 98–99, 114
Motor coordination, 48, 63
Mulder, R., 44
Murphy, A., 46
Musculature:
    nonspeech, 8–11
    speech, 8–11, 32, 57, 83–84, 124

Neill, A., 66, 67
Netsell, R., 57
Neurological disorders, 110
Neuromuscular skills, 35
Niebuhr, R., 152

Off-line analysis, 116–17
Ogburn, R. S., 146, 151
On-line analysis, 116, 117–20
Onset, of stuttering, 11, 27
    case study, 158–63

Onufrak, J., 146, 151
Orientation, to therapy situation, 169
Overarticulation, 32

Parallel-process, 8–9
Parent(s):
    attitudes, towards therapy, 79
    counseling of, 15, 18, 32, 37, 43, 44, 45,
        64–67, 85
    interview procedure, 154–57, 158,
        159–61, 163
    reaction, to stuttering, 76
    role, in speech development, 40
    role, in therapy, 48, 50–51, 85–86
    standards of, 23–24, 25, 44–45, 67, 140
    supportive role, 99
Parent-child interaction, 46, 47, 50, 77–78
Part-word repetition, 55, 83, 93
Passivity, 25, 36
Pausing, between syllables, 7, 9, 11
Peabody Picture Vocabulary Test, 48
Peers, interaction with, 78, 103
Perception:
    by listener, 7–11, 18, 25–26, 124
    by parents, 44–48
    by stutterer, 26, 61, 118, 120–21, 122,
        141–42
    by therapist, 83, 120–21, 124
Perkins, W., 10, 16
Perkins, W. H., 3, 16, 144
Personal characteristics, of therapist,
    148–50, 164–67
Peters, T., 28, 147
Phonetic placement procedure, 32
Placebo effect, 86, 87
Play therapy, 46, 50
Prins, D., 16, 25, 26, 64, 80
Problem solving approach to therapy, 6–7,
    18
Professional development, of therapist,
    167–69
Professional responsibility, of therapist, 65,
    104
Psyche philosophy, of stuttering, 146
Psychological aspects of stuttering, 3–4, 8,
    11, 14, 35–37, 62, 80, 87–88
Psychological services, referral to, 35,
    36–37, 45, 65, 99, 103
Psychosocial aspects of stuttering, 3–4, 8,
    10, 16, 36, 48, 103–4, 136
Psychosocial problems, of adolescence,
    90–91, 99
Psychotherapy, 108
Publications, self-help, 44, 45

Quantification of stuttering physiology, 61
Quarrington, R., 16, 92
Questioning, during interview, 23–25,
    154–57

Ramig, P., 145, 146
Reading:
    to child, 53–54
    oral, 24, 29, 33, 89
    problems, 64, 104
Recipe approach, 6
Rees, N., 52
Reevaluation:
    of adolescent stutterer, 104
    of child stutterer, 47, 49
Referral(s):
    by employer, 110
    to other professionals, 35, 36–37, 64–65
    to psychological services, 35, 36–37, 45,
        65, 99, 103
    for speech therapy, 37–38
Reinforcement:
    positive, 82, 85, 87, 98, 127–28, 129
    of stuttering-associated behavior, 9–10
Relapse, 86, 131–32, 143, 144–45
Relaxation, of speech mechanism, 84
Release, from speech posture, 62, 87–89,
    125
Remediation:
    adults, 108–37
    older children and teenagers, 70–106
    young children, 41–68
Repetition:
    part-word, 55, 83, 93
    of speech posture, 98
    of syllables, 7, 10, 11, 79, 117
    words, 7–8, 48
Response, differential, of listener, 10–11
Reynolds, G., 3
Rieber, R. W., 94
Right-to-know, 22
Robinson, F., 7, 27, 103
Role playing, 130
Rosenbek, J., 110
Rothenberg, M., 98
Runyan, C., 151
Ryan, B., 142

Schery, T., 47
School authorities, 64, 104–5
Seebach, M., 12, 31
Self-confidence, 108–9
Self-image, 16–17, 38, 50, 78
Sensitivity, of therapist, 119, 126, 165
Shaefer, C. E., 66
Shames, G., 82, 91, 145, 147
Shapiro, A. I., 12
Shapiro, A., 87
Sheehan, J., 35, 36, 91, 102, 142
Shoemaker, D., 9, 27, 59, 81
Shriberg, L., 20, 32
Siblings, interaction with stutterer, 51–52,
    53
Siegel, G., 115
Silverman, F., 16

Skinner, B. F., 10
Skolnick, M. L., 26
Social maturity, of child, 70, 86
Social withdrawal, 103
Soma philosophy, of stuttering, 146
Sound:
  syllable-initial, 62
  word-initial, 62, 63, 88
Sound production, anxiety concerning, 49
Sound prolongation, 7, 10, 11, 37, 48–49,
  54, 79, 83, 117, 124, 127
Sound repetition, 7, 10, 117
Speaking rate, 29
Speaking situations, 27, 38, 88, 99–101,
  103, 111, 144
Speaking strategies, 18, 62, 123, 125, 128,
  132
Speech. See also Articulation
  descriptive phrases, 61
  hard-easy concept, 50–51, 61, 73
  initiation, 49, 50
  microscopic analysis, 22
Speech development, parental role in, 40
Speech discrimination test, 30
Speech disfluency. See also Stuttering
  between-word, 8, 29
  and delayed language, 48
  frequency, 29, 55, 82
  listener's perception, 7–8
  marginal, 112
  normal limits, 44
  within-word, 8, 11, 15, 29, 38, 47, 82, 83,
    144
Speech fluency:
  basal level, 74
  causes, 145–48
  disruptor, 74–77
  evaluation, 28–30
  individual differences in, 15–16
  initiating gestures, 145
  voice onset time during, 31
Speech-language pathologist:
  attitudes towards, 20
  beliefs and expectations, 87
  client relationship, 87, 95, 119, 126, 129
  credibility, 46
  imitation, 60, 81–82
  knowledge of stuttering, 14, 20, 135–36
  orientation to stuttering, 2–7, 139
  personal characteristics, 148–50
  professional development, 167–69
  self-analysis, 164–65
  supportive role, 87, 93, 98–99, 113, 126
  training, 20, 64, 111–12, 151, 167–70
Speech mechanism closure, 57
Speech model, 54, 60, 88
Speech musculature, 8–11, 32, 57, 83–84,
  124
Speech physiology, 3–4, 7, 11–14, 61–62,
  98, 124, 126–27

Speech posture:
  release from, 62, 87–89, 125
  repetition, 98
Speech production:
  analogies, 56–60, 84
  child's understanding of, 56–61
  demonstration of, 60–61, 84, 96–98, 126,
    129
  description of, 142–43
  homogenization, 146–47
  physiological basis, 98
  strategies, 18, 62, 123, 125, 128, 132
  temporal expansion, 146–47
  visualization, 60–61
Spock, B., 47
Sports, organized, 78
Spriestersbach, D., 10
Starbuck, H., 25, 64, 80
Starkweather, C., 125
Stevens, K., 26
Stimulation, of language behavior, 33
Stocker, B., 51, 101
Stocker Probe Test, 101
Story-telling, by child, 33, 50
Stress, 46, 146
Stromsta, C., 12
Student-clinicians, 168
Stutterer. See also client
  attitudes towards stuttering, 9, 108–9
  awareness of stuttering, 10, 26, 47, 54,
    71, 72–74, 120, 131, 141
  definition, 15–17, 108
  individuality of, 4–5, 7, 15–16, 33, 35, 107
  marginally disfluent, 112
  perception of stuttering, 26, 61, 118,
    120–21, 122, 141–42
  self-image, 16–17, 38, 50, 78
  variation in therapy response, 4–5
Stuttering. See also Speech disfluency
  in adolescents, 69–106
  in adults, 25–26, 106–37
  behavioral composite, 3, 8, 13, 29–30,
    81–82, 134
  behavioral description, 3, 13
  in children, 11–14, 34, 44–60
  definition, 11, 39
  developmental stages, 11–14, 80
  duration, 120, 121
  easily recognizable, 124
  etiology, 27–28, 144, 146, 147–48
  evaluation 8, 20–39, 42, 44–60, 83, 101,
    139–40
  frequency, 133
  increased, 120–21
  onset, 11, 27, 158–63
  perception, 7–11, 18, 24, 25–26, 61, 83,
    118, 120–21, 122, 124, 141–42
  physiological aspects, 3–4, 7, 11–14,
    61–62, 124, 126–27

psychological aspects, 3–4, 8, 11–14,
    36–37, 62, 80, 87–88
psychosocial aspects of, 3–4, 8, 10, 16,
    36, 48
relapse, 86, 131–32, 143, 144–45
Supportive role:
    of parents, 99
    of speech-language pathologist, 87, 93,
        98–99, 113, 126
Syllable-initial sound, 62
Syllable pauses, 7, 9, 11
Syllable repetition, 7, 10, 11, 79, 117
Syracuse University, 42, 62

Talking:
    with child, 53, 78, 85
    encouragement of, 89
Tape recorder:
    audio, 21–22, 96–98, 115, 118, 141
    video, 60, 115, 141
Teasing, of child stutterer, 51–52
Telephone, use in speech practice, 99,
    100–101, 130
Tension, 8–11, 47, 48–49, 83–84, 119, 124
Test(s):
    Ammon's Quick Test, 48
    Peabody Picture Vocabulary Test, 48
    speech discrimination, 30
    Stocker Probe, 101
    Vineland Test of Social Maturity, 48
Therapist. See Speech-language pathologist
Therapy. See also Group therapy
    attitudes towards, 63–64, 70, 79, 111
    consistency of approach, 148
    contraindication, 32, 44, 104
    direct, 41, 42
    discontinuation, 63–64, 86–87, 92,
        133–34
    failure, 93–94, 170–71
    follow-up sessions, 134–35
    frequency and duration, 113–14
    future directions, 150–52
    history, 93–94, 108
    indirect, 15, 41, 42
    initiation, 96
    parental role, 48, 50–51, 85–86
    play, 46, 50
    practice assignments, 63, 89–90, 112, 131
    problem solving approach, 6–7, 18
    prognosis, 35, 36, 79, 80, 113, 135
    referral for, 37–38
    trial, 38, 114, 115
    variation in response, 4–5
Therapy procedures, 5
    for adolescent, 90–106
    for adult, 109–37
    for child, 40–68
Tone screening, 30

Transition, articulatory, 62–63, 87, 88,
    97–98, 123, 125
Trial therapy, 38, 114, 115
Turner, P., 59

Uncooperativeness, in therapy, 92
Ushijima, T., 12, 31, 61, 83

Vaillant, G., 36
Van Naerssen, E., 33
Van Riper, C., 5, 6, 7, 21, 36, 44, 46, 50,
    51, 52, 53, 62, 64, 74, 77, 84, 94, 102,
    116, 125, 129, 148, 149
Variability:
    sound-to-sound, 145
    of speech production, 146
Verbal expression, of child stutterer, 52–53,
    77
Verbal interaction, 53
Vineland Test of Social Maturity, 48
Visualization, of speech production, 60–61,
    97
Vocabulary development, 16, 54
Vocabulary recognition, 48
Vocal nodules, 31
Vocal pitch, changes in, 14, 31, 147
Vocal quality, 29, 79, 124
Vocal tract:
    closure, 57
    muscle contraction, 9
Voice disorders, 30–32
Voice onset time (VOT), 3

Webster, R., 84, 123, 147
Willemain, T., 26
Williams, D., 10, 11, 16
Williams, D. E., 3, 6, 9, 15, 26, 42, 44, 50,
    51, 52, 62, 73, 87, 144
Wingate, M. E., 8, 28, 72, 121, 129
Winitz, H., 16, 32
Winn, M., 54, 78
Withdrawal, social, 103
Word-initial sound, 62, 63, 88
Word repetition, 7–8, 48
Word substitution, 80
Writing, as sound transition analogy,
    62–63, 98

Yairi, E., 16

Zilbergeld, B., 144
Zimmerman, G., 83
Zwitman, D., 76